Save your GALLBLADDER naturally

(and what to do if you've already lost it)

By

Sandra Cabot MD
and
Margaret Jasinska ND

www.liverdoctor.com

www.sandracabot.com

The information and procedures contained in this book are based upon the research and the professional experiences of the authors.

The recommendations in this book are not intended as a substitute for consulting with your own physician. All persons with gallbladder problems should remain under the care of their personal physician.

Published in the United States of America by SCB International Inc

PO Box 5070, Glendale Phoenix AZ 85312-5070

Telephone 1-888-755-4837

Distributed in the UK & Europe by

Roundhouse Group, Maritime House,

Basin Road North, Hove BN41 1WR

T. 01273 704 962 F. 01273 704 963

W. www.roundhousegroup.co.uk

E. alan@roundhousegroup.co.uk

Internet address:

www.liverdoctor.com

www.sandracabot.com

ISBN 978-1-936609-16-1

Contents

About the Authors

Sandra Cabot MD

Dr Sandra Cabot is the author of twenty five books on health including the famous Liver Cleansing Diet book which has sold over 2 million copies and is translated into 6 languages. She graduated with Honors in Medicine and Surgery in 1975 from Adelaide University, South Australia. During the 1980s Sandra spent considerable time working in the Department of Obstetrics and Gynecology in a large missionary hospital in the Himalayan foothills of India.

Dr Cabot has lectured for the American Liver Foundation, The Primary Biliary Cirrhosis Society and The Hepatitis C Council of Australia where she was the protagonist in the great debate "Does the liver need a good cleanse?"

Dr Cabot is involved in raising funds for women's refuges in Australia and is an Angel Flight pilot for disadvantaged patients living in rural Australia.

Margaret Jasinska ND

Margaret Jasinska is a naturopath with more than sixteen years of clinical experience. Margaret has co-authored seven books with Dr Cabot. She divides her time between seeing patients at Dr Cabot's clinic, writing and researching new developments in health and medicine.

Margaret's main area of interest is in digestive and immune system disorders. She greatly enjoys empowering individuals to improve their health by giving them the tools and knowledge to lead healthier lives. Health and wellness is a great passion and hobby of hers.

She practices what she preaches and her two dogs, Henry and Dayna, are both on a gluten and dairy free diet.

Introduction

Between ten and 15 percent of Americans are affected by gallbladder disease at some point in their life. Gallbladder surgery is one of the most commonly performed hospital procedures. Gallbladder disease can be painful and frightening, yet too many people are rushed off to surgery to have their gallbladder removed, when in most cases there are safe and natural alternatives.

Too few people realize it is possible to dissolve gallstones and restore a healthy gallbladder in the majority of cases

What if there was a natural way to dissolve stones, keep your gallbladder and avoid the risks of surgery? There is; please keep reading and we will explain how.

Gallbladder surgery is a lucrative industry; thousands of gallbladders are removed each year. That would be alright if the surgery was absolutely critical and there was no other alternative, and if the surgery fixed all of the patient's problems and they felt fantastic afterwards. Unfortunately it is usually not the case. In the vast majority of instances, the gallbladder could have been saved if the patient was given the right advice. Conventional advice states to avoid eating greasy, oily food. That is really only five percent of the solution. So many other factors can lead to malfunction of the gallbladder and stones, yet most patients are never fully informed of them.

The other problem is that **a significant number of patients who have had their gallbladder removed continue to suffer with pain and digestive problems.** Sometimes these symptoms are even worse after surgery. According to a study published in the British Journal of General Practice it was found that having the gallbladder surgically removed does not always relieve upper abdominal pain.[1] This is true even in those who have proven gallstones. This is because removing the gallbladder doesn't address the original condition that caused stones to form in the first place. Along with continued pain, people who have had their gallbladder removed are at increased risk of certain liver diseases.

Clearly the medical model of "when in doubt, cut it out" is not the best solution for most patients. We want to tell you the real cause of gallstones and other gallbladder disorders and give you the tools to heal yourself.

In this book we expose the most common myths surrounding the gallbladder and give you the true facts. For example:

Myth - You need to follow a low fat diet to prevent or shrink gallstones.

Fact - The opposite is true. A low fat diet actually encourages the formation of stones for three reasons:

1. Excess carbohydrate is converted into fat in your liver

2. Low fat diets promote bile stasis

3. Gluten can interfere with gallbladder contractions;

thus all three factors promote gallstones. You need to eat some fat in order to flush the gallbladder clean and avoid stagnation of bile. Sugar is a bigger problem for the gallbladder than fat is.

Myth - People with gallbladder disease should avoid saturated fat.

Fact - Many commonly consumed saturated fats are composed of short and medium chain fatty acids. These fats do not require bile for their digestion therefore do not place a strain on the gallbladder. For example coconut oil and ghee are saturated fats predominantly composed of medium and short chain fatty acids respectively, and are okay to eat.

Myth - A gallbladder flush is the best way to get rid of gallstones.

Fact - A gallbladder flush is not for everyone. If you are already in pain, it can make the pain significantly worse, and even lead to an emergency trip to hospital where you'd likely return without your gallbladder.

Myth - It doesn't matter if your gallbladder is removed. It's not an important organ and you can be perfectly healthy without it.

Fact - Yes, it's true that you can survive quite well without a gallbladder, but you are at greater risk of developing certain liver conditions. You will also have impaired fat digestion and probable deficiency of fat soluble nutrients such as vitamins including vitamins D, K, E and A, as well as essential fatty acids.

Myth - Having your gallbladder removed will stop the pain and then you can eat whatever you like.

Fact - This is not the case for many people. Some people experience even worse symptoms after their gallbladder is taken out. Either way, removing the gallbladder does not address the underlying metabolic abnormalities that caused a person to develop stones in the first place.

Myth - You can't do a liver detox if you don't have a gallbladder.

Fact - Yes, you can do a liver detox and it is critical to take good care of your liver in order to avoid developing stones within the liver and other liver disorders.

Myth - It is normal and expected that you'll have digestive problems such as irritable bowel syndrome or diarrhea after having your gallbladder removed and it's just something you'll have to live with.

Fact - No it isn't. There are ways to ensure good digestion and help you be symptom free and we will show you how.

Gallstones are not always caused by an abnormality of the gallbladder; they are caused by problems with the liver and digestive system, which promote the production of unhealthy bile, which is then more likely to form stones. Digestive problems can also interfere with the ability of the gallbladder to contract, thus further encouraging stone formation and inflammation of the gallbladder.

The key to healing your gallbladder lies with fixing your liver and digestive system, as well as overcoming nutritional deficiencies

Keep reading and you'll discover what really causes gallstones, and how you can prevent or treat them naturally and safely.

A word of caution

The recommendations in this book are of a very general nature and may not be appropriate for every single reader. It is crucial that you consult with your own doctor in regards to any medical problems or symptoms you are experiencing. Please make sure you get an accurate diagnosis and do not solely rely on the information in this book.

Not every case of gallbladder disease can be healed with natural remedies. Sometimes surgery is the most appropriate and the safest option. If you experience pain or other distressing symptoms, please do not delay consulting with your doctor. The recommendations in this book are designed as an adjunct to advice you receive from your own doctor, not a replacement.

Case study

I will never forget a patient of mine who was already in her 70s when she first consulted me. She was troubled by chronic but intermittent pain over the area of her liver (right upper quadrant of the abdomen). This pain was due to cysts in her liver as well as cysts in her bile ducts. She had had her gallbladder removed in her 40s, because of stones and sludge. Notwithstanding, the reduction in her symptoms was modest and she continued to have intermittent pain. Over the years she developed more liver cysts and had some stones form in her bile ducts, even though her gallbladder was removed.

These recurrent stones caused temporary and painful blockages in her bile ducts and this increased the size of her liver cysts. This is not surprising, as blockages lead to an increase in pressure in the ducts and pressure leads to swelling in the tubes, which can lead to cysts. She had gained excess weight since her gallbladder was removed.

I thought to myself – "This lady is a real challenge, as the surgeons had not been able to help her."

Once I examined her and took her history I could see that she was very dehydrated and had red palms. Red palms are a common sign of liver disease. Her skin and her eyes had a yellowish or sallow complexion and her tongue was coated with a green-white colored layer. She did not drink very much water and her diet was lacking in raw fruits and vegetables. Most of her food was cooked. She did eat vegetables, which was one positive thing, but they were generally over cooked. She did not eat fruit every day and did not take vitamin C, so she was sure to have a vitamin C deficiency.

This elderly lady was a prime example of the need to take care of your liver and bile ducts, even after your gallbladder is removed. Her surgeon had told her that she "could eat anything and everything now that her gallbladder was removed". How incorrect is that!

Because she had not known how to take care of her bile ducts, she had suffered needlessly for many years. Well that was about to change, as she was going to start supporting her gallbladder and bile ducts with the right diet and nutritional supplements. By supporting the production of healthy bile by the liver cells we can keep the bile ducts healthy and avoid the formation of more stones in the bile ducts.

Even if you have had your gallbladder out, we encourage you to support your liver in its major functions of bile manufacture and detoxification.

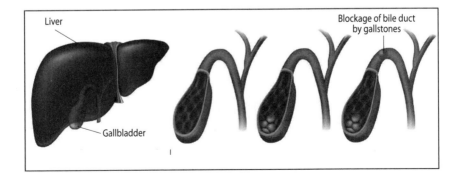

Chapter One

Types of gallbladder disorders covered in this book

This book primarily focuses on gallstones, since they are by far the most common condition affecting the gallbladder. However, there are several other gallbladder conditions that we have covered in this book. The vast majority of dietary guidelines we offer for gallstones are equally applicable for other gallbladder conditions.

Other conditions affecting the gallbladder include:

- **Cholecystitis** - this refers to inflammation of the gallbladder. It often goes hand in hand with gallstones but may precede gallstones by several years. The metabolic problems that lead to gallstones also promote inflammation of the gallbladder. Therefore the remedies for gallstones and cholecystitis are mostly the same. Sometimes a bacterial infection of the gallbladder can cause cholecystitis.

- **Bile sludge** - this is a common finding on ultrasound and usually precedes gallstones. The bile has started to thicken abnormally and is highly likely to soon form stones.

- **Gallbladder polyps** - these are nodule like growths that can form in the gallbladder.

- **Thickened walls of the gallbladder** - it is common to notice on an ultrasound report that the gallbladder walls are thickened.

- **Calcified gallbladder** (*sometimes called porcelain gallbladder*) - where the walls of the gallbladder have become calcified and very hard.

- **Gallbladder cancer**

- **Autoimmune diseases of the biliary ducts**, including primary biliary cirrhosis and sclerosing cholangitis.

We cover these conditions in chapter ten, however the vast majority of recommendations in this book are equally applicable to all gallbladder and biliary conditions. This is because our aim in healing your gallbladder is to correct the problems with your liver, digestive system and metabolism that created the gallbladder problem in the first place.

Incidence of gallbladder disease

Gallbladder conditions are incredibly common. An acute gallbladder attack is actually the most common hospital admission for a digestive condition. Apart from cataract surgery, gallbladder surgery is one of the most commonly performed operations in the USA. Gallstones are the most common gallbladder pathology and they occur in roughly 10 to 15 percent of the population.

What are gallstones?

Gallstones form when bile stored in the gallbladder hardens into stone-like objects. This process usually takes years. In fact the estimated growth rate of gallstones is approximately 2 millimetres per year.[2]

Normal bile is made up of a combination of water, cholesterol, lecithin, other fats, bile acids, bilirubin, waste products and proteins. If the concentration of cholesterol in the bile becomes too high, relative to bile acids, cholesterol can precipitate out and form stones. Gallstones can be as small as a grain of sand or as large as a golf ball.

There are several types of gallstones:

- **Cholesterol stones**
- **Pigment stones** - these are formed from calcium bilirubinate (a component of bilirubin) and appear black or brown.
- **Mixed stones** - some people have both types of stones in their gallbladder

Cholesterol stones are by far the most common type, accounting for 80 percent of all gallstones. They are made of hardened cholesterol and look yellow-green in color.

Pigment stones are made of bilirubin (breakdown product of red blood cells), they are smaller and dark colored. Pigment stones are more common in developing nations and are usually the result of liver infections, cirrhosis of the liver, hemolytic anemia or other metabolic disorders. Because pigment stones are uncommon and usually caused by a serious illness, we have not discussed the treatment of these stones in this book.

Risk factors for gallbladder disease

Who is most likely to suffer with gallbladder disease?

Women are far more likely to develop gallstones than men, and this is mostly because of the effect of female hormones. Medical students are taught to suspect gallstones if the patient is:

- Fat
- Fair
- Female
- Fertile (meaning before menopause)
- Forty, as this is the typical age when gallstones first present.

Gallstones are more likely to occur in Western European, Hispanic and Native American people compared with Eastern European, Japanese and African American people.

Being overweight increases the risk of getting gallstones by approximately 80 percent. High doses of synthetic hormones in oral contraceptives and hormone replacement therapy increase the risk of gallstones because estrogen increases the amount of cholesterol secreted into bile. This makes the bile thicker and more likely to form stones. For this same reason, gallbladder problems sometimes first manifest themselves during pregnancy.

Other factors that increase the risk of gallbladder disease

Here are some other factors that raise the risk of gallbladder disease:

- Syndrome X (also known as insulin resistance or metabolic syndrome)
- Diabetes
- Obesity [3.]
- Females are more likely to develop gallbladder disease than males and women who have had several children are at highest risk (due to the extremely high levels of hormones in the bloodstream during pregnancy).
- Hypothyroidism (under active thyroid gland). This condition usually causes elevated cholesterol, a reduced metabolic rate and slowed digestion. People with an under active thyroid are also more likely to suffer with sluggish bile flow and delayed emptying of the gallbladder. [4.]
- Food intolerance or food sensitivities. This is a very common yet under-recognized cause of gallbladder disease. Food sensitivities impair healthy digestion and can reduce the ability of the gallbladder to contract and empty fully. Stasis of bile within the gallbladder promotes the formation of sludge and the eventual formation of gallstones.
- Low stomach acid (hypochlorhydria). This goes hand in hand with indigestion and food intolerance. Many people spend much of their lives taking antacid medication that reduces stomach acid. Common brands include Nexium, Protonix and Zantac.
- Gluten intolerance/celiac disease. There is a strong association between this condition and gallbladder disease.
- Having a family history of gallbladder disease.
- Rapid weight loss. If you lose weight extremely quickly, where does the fat go? Your hard working liver will break it down because it is the main fat burning organ in your body. Then the fat will

be secreted into your gallbladder as a component of bile. Bile can then become super saturated with fat and raise the risk of stones forming. Alternatively stones that were already in your gallbladder can grow bigger.

- Estrogen in contraceptives or hormone replacement therapy. Estrogen increases the amount of cholesterol in bile and that makes stones more likely to form. Women naturally have much more estrogen in their bodies than men and this is why they suffer from gallbladder disease more frequently than men.

- Very low fat diets. Every time you eat fat, hormone signals are sent to your gallbladder prompting it to contract and empty its contents into your small intestine. If you don't eat enough fat, old bile will stay inside your gallbladder too long and that raises the risk of stones. It is important to eat adequate healthy, unprocessed fat in order to keep your bile moving and keep your gallbladder clean.

- People with high cholesterol and high triglycerides in their blood are at increased risk of gallstones.

- Cholesterol lowering drugs raise the risk of gallstones; particularly statins and clofibrate.

- Having a fatty liver or sluggish, overworked liver significantly raises the risk of developing gallstones. In fact they are almost inevitable.

- People with indigestion, bloating, heartburn, reflux, flatulence or burping are more prone to developing gallbladder disease.

- High alcohol intake.

- Binge eating or eating excessively large meals. Eating more food than your digestive organs can handle is a risk factor for developing gallstones and a major risk factor for getting a gallbladder attack and emergency trip to the hospital if you already have gallstones.

- The antibiotic ceftriaxone.

- Diets high in sugar or other carbohydrate rich foods, junk food and deep fried food.

- Constipation.
- Diets lacking fiber.
- Inflammatory bowel disease (Crohn's disease and ulcerative colitis)
- Infection in the stomach with the bacteria Helicobacter pylori raises the risk of cholecystitis (inflammation of the gallbladder). [5] The presence of this bacteria also seems to be associated with cancer of the gallbladder or biliary tract. [6]

Helicobacter pylori is a very common bacterial infection that raises the risk of stomach ulcers and stomach cancer. It is important not to have an overgrowth of this bacteria in your digestive system because it creates chronic inflammation, which can eventually lead to serious disease.

The most effective way to eradicate Helicobacter pylori is to improve the health and function of your digestive system. Parasites and pathogenic organisms are attracted to a sick and dysfunctional digestive tract. You need to make your digestive system healthy and inhospitable to harmful bugs. There are also excellent herbal products designed specifically to eradicate harmful microbes from the digestive system.

Symptoms of gallbladder dysfunction

Gallstones are incredibly common and it is estimated that in 80 percent of cases they are asymptomatic and the person doesn't realize they have them. In truth, gallstones always cause symptoms, but sometimes they are very subtle and a person does not realize the source of the problem.

The classic symptom most people associate with gallstones is pain or discomfort in the right upper quadrant of the abdomen (just behind the lowest right rib) after a meal. It is important to be aware of the other more subtle symptoms of an unhappy gallbladder that you would not normally associate with this condition. Sometimes they can be early warning signs that bigger problems are just around the corner.

The most common signs and symptoms of gallbladder dysfunction include:

- Indigestion, particularly after eating rich fatty meals or dairy products
- Abdominal bloating or a feeling of excessive fullness after meals.
- Reflux or heartburn, also known as GERD
- Diarrhea or loose, urgent stools after some foods
- Abdominal cramps or other pain after a meal
- Discomfort behind the right shoulder blade, or top of the right shoulder
- Moody, irritable disposition
- Low tolerance to alcohol
- Sweating feet or excess sweating in the body in general
- Bad breath and coated tongue
- Fatigue after eating.

Symptoms of a gallbladder attack

You may experience some or all of the above symptoms to varying degrees if you have gallbladder disease. However, a gallbladder attack produces far more extreme symptoms. A gallbladder attack can occur if a gallstone gets trapped in the neck of the gallbladder, or gets stuck in a bile duct. This can inhibit the normal flow of bile and lead to a buildup of pressure within the biliary system. Spasms of the bile ducts can also lead to pain and discomfort.

Symptoms of a gallbladder attack can be extreme and can lead to an emergency trip to the hospital. It is also possible to have a gallbladder attack when no stones can be found in the gallbladder. These symptoms can be caused by inflammation to the walls of the gallbladder (cholecystitis), or gallbladder sludge or a stone trapped within a bile duct inside the liver.

Symptoms of a gallbladder attack may include the following:

- Intense pain in the right upper quadrant of the abdomen (just behind the lowest rib on the right). The area can be so tender that it takes your breath away if you apply pressure to it.
- Nausea that may lead to vomiting
- Sweating
- Flatulence (intestinal gas)
- Diarrhea
- Belching (burping)
- A fever
- Pain may radiate to the right shoulder blade, or between the shoulder blades
- The pain may be so intense that it becomes impossible to walk unless hunched over
- The pain may come and go or it may be constant.

The symptoms of a gallbladder attack usually last between one and four hours

It most frequently occurs after a heavy meal, high in fat; typically after dinner. Therefore most gallbladder attacks occur at night.

What causes the pain of a gallbladder attack?

Meals that contain a lot of fat, or large meals cause forceful gallbladder contractions. If the gallbladder is inflamed, which is almost always the case with long standing gallstones, powerful contractions can hurt a lot. Even if no stones are present in the gallbladder, powerful contractions can hurt if the gallbladder contracts forcefully.

The intense pain of a gallbladder attack and associated symptoms can be caused by a stone that left the gallbladder and became trapped in a bile duct on its way to the small intestine. The symptoms of a gallbladder attack can also be caused by a back up of bile within the gallbladder that causes it to swell, leading to discomfort (there may or may not be stones present in the gallbladder). A trapped stone, or a build up of bile can also lead to spasms of the bile ducts, which causes more pain.

An inflamed gallbladder (cholecystitis) can produce the symptoms of a gallbladder attack, with or without the presence of stones. Sometimes the inflammation is due to a bacterial infection within the gallbladder or bile ducts, but chronic inflammation can also be caused by food allergies.

Of course, the symptoms of a gallbladder attack are very similar to symptoms of several other serious medical conditions, so if you are in intense or regular pain, please do not assume that it's just your gallbladder. It is essential to see your local doctor and obtain an accurate diagnosis.

Chapter Two

The natural treatment of gallstones

This is where we show you our seven point plan for restoring the health of your gallbladder. These recommendations are applicable for people wishing to dissolve gallstones, prevent gallstones or heal an otherwise dysfunctional or inflamed gallbladder that is causing pain or discomfort.

The cornerstone of this treatment is to heal your liver and digestive function.

This makes perfect sense because your liver is the organ that makes bile and an overloaded liver that produces unhealthy bile is the fundamental cause of gallstones.

Several factors can be responsible for overloading the liver; some of them are dietary, and others are related to problems with the digestive tract.

Natural remedies take time, so you will need to have some patience.

Your gallstones did not develop overnight; they have probably been there for at least ten years. Therefore it is realistic to expect natural remedies to take many months to a couple of years to dissolve gallstones.

However, if you follow our guidelines, you can expect to feel better within weeks. Our immediate aim is to help prevent a gallbladder attack and keep you out of hospital, so that the natural remedies have long enough to work on dissolving the stones. I'm sure you won't mind being patient with dissolving the stones if you are relieved to be free of chronic pain and indigestion.

Depending on your specific scenario, you may still experience gallbladder attacks while following our program; but they should be significantly milder and less frequent. If you are highly motivated and follow our advice to the letter, most of you should be rewarded with a much healthier gallbladder and avoidance of gallbladder surgery.

The majority of the strategies for gallbladder disease are diet changes; this makes sense because it is unhealthy or inappropriate diet choices that lead to gallbladder problems.

The seven essential strategies for treating gallbladder disease

1. Keep the bile fluid and keep it moving - ie. prevent bile stasis and bile sludge

An abnormal composition of bile is what promotes gallstone formation in the first place, therefore correcting this abnormality is the key to dissolving gallstones and preventing their recurrence. The underlying cause of cholesterol stones in the gallbladder is bile that is overly concentrated in cholesterol. We refer to this as cholesterol super-saturation of bile. There is too much cholesterol in the bile relative to bile acids, therefore the cholesterol cannot dissolve properly and it precipitates out, creating stones.

Therefore what we want to do is make your bile thinner, increase the amount of bile acids relative to cholesterol, and help your gallbladder to contract properly so that bile doesn't remain trapped inside too long.

One of the simplest ways to prevent your bile from getting too thick is to drink plenty of water each day. Many people walk around in a chronic state of dehydration; getting so busy each day that they forget to drink all day. Coffee, tea and alcohol are all diuretics, which worsen dehydration. Please drink approximately 67 ounces (two litres) of fluid each day, which can be a combination of water, herbal tea and vegetable juice.

The other way to prevent bile becoming too thick is to reduce the amount of cholesterol in your body. See point number five for information on how to do that. You must also increase the amount of bile acids in your bile. This will make the bile thinner, thus helping to dissolve any stones inside the gallbladder, and helping to prevent new ones forming. See point number four in this chapter for information on how to do this.

Do not follow a low fat diet

A common recommendation for anyone with gallstones is to follow a low fat diet. This is the worst thing you can do and it can make your gallstones much worse. People are told to avoid fat because eating too much fat can cause powerful gallbladder contractions and that will make your pain much worse. It is certainly important to avoid unhealthy fats, as described on page 53, and to avoid eating too much fat in one go.

People with gallbladder disease are also told to avoid fat in their diet in the mistaken belief that eating fat raises blood cholesterol levels. This is not the case; carbohydrate rich foods are the worst culprits when it comes to raising cholesterol. We have explained this fully in point number five.

It is important to include some good fats with each meal in order to keep bile flowing through your gallbladder. Eating some fat promotes your gallbladder to contract and squeeze the bile inside it out into your common bile duct and eventually into your small intestine. If you do not eat enough fat, the bile will remain in your gallbladder for too long. Old bile will stay in your gallbladder, and the longer it stays there, the more concentrated it will become. This means you will have bile stasis in your gallbladder and that is a recipe for gallstones. Also, if you are not eating much fat, by default you will be consuming more carbohydrate. Your liver will convert much of the carbohydrate into triglycerides and cholesterol, which further thicken your bile.

So as you can see, eating some fat each day is extremely important for keeping your gallbladder clean and flushing fresh bile through your gallbladder.

2. The best foods and herbs for the gallbladder

Cholerectics and cholagogues - foods and herbs that promote bile production and secretion

Just by improving your liver and digestive function and normalizing the composition of your bile, you should be able to dissolve your gallstones in time. However there are specific herbs and nutrients that help to speed up that process.

- A **choleretic** is a substance that increases bile production and secretion in the liver.
- A **cholagogue** is a substance that increases bile secretion by the gallbladder, thereby promoting more bile to reach the small intestine.

There are various foods and herbs with these properties. They also have a cleansing effect on the liver and gallbladder, and help to ease indigestion and promote a healthier digestive tract.

A choleretic mainly works on the liver and a cholagogue mainly works on the gallbladder. However, many foods and herbs actually have both of these actions. It is not important to remember these terms, but you may come across them if you do your own reading about herbs for the liver and gallbladder. Now you know what the terms mean.

Bitter foods and herbs

The specific foods and herbs for the gallbladder are predominantly bitter tasting ones. This is no coincidence. Bitter substances stimulate the nerve endings of the vagus nerve on your tongue, which triggers the secretion of digestive enzymes and juices further along your digestive tract.

Basically bitter foods and herbs turn on your digestive system and prepare it for food. They promote the production and secretion of bile, helping to keep it moving through your liver and gallbladder. You have probably heard of Swedish Bitters, available from health food stores and designed to be consumed before meals.

Traditionally a salad made of bitter leaves is eaten as an entree or aperitif, to help prime the digestive system for the heavier meal to follow.

Best foods for the gallbladder

Beet leaves

Dandelion leaves

Chicory leaves

Endive

Radicchio lettuce

Beets

Fresh mint leaves

Globe artichoke

Radishes - *both red radishes and the long, huge white radish (daikon radish)*

Lemons

Limes

Arugula *(rocket)*

Kale

Watercress

Basil

Cabbage

Try to include these vegetables and fruits in your diet as often as possible. They promote the production and secretion of bile, and in this way have a cleansing effect on your gallbladder. They can be added to salads or cooked. You could steam these vegetables or include them in soups, stews and casseroles.

Raw vegetable juice for the gallbladder

You will find this same juice recipe in the section of this book describing the gallbladder flush, as it is a helpful part of the preparation for doing a flush. However we encourage you to drink this vegetable juice regularly, whether you decide to do a gallbladder flush or not. Try to drink one glass of this juice every day, or as often as possible.

Ingredients

1 large beet

8 large beet leaves

8 chicory or endive leaves

2 stalks celery

¼ red onion

1 large carrot

2 red radishes

1 small apple

Method

Pass all ingredients through a juice extractor and drink. Sometimes it is hard to find fresh beet leaves. The beet may look good but the leaves are wilted and completely dead. You may also have difficulty finding chicory or endive. Beet leaves are particularly beneficial for the gallbladder. Chicory and endive are very bitter and all bitter foods stimulate the release of bile from the gallbladder. This helps to prevent bile stagnation in the gallbladder.

Many greengrocers sell fresh beet leaves, chicory and endive, so it may be worth a drive to the next suburb to find a good greengrocer You could also ask your local greengrocer to get these vegetables in for you.

Alternatively if you have a little vegetable patch at home, these leafy vegetables are extremely easy to grow, as long as you keep the snails away and water them regularly. Both of us grow several varieties of vegetables and herbs in our home gardens and it is such a luxury to have fresh produce each day for salads and juicing.

Green goodness soup for the gallbladder

This soup is rich in those vegetables specifically beneficial for your liver and gallbladder. This is one idea on how to use these vegetables; you could also add them to stews or casseroles or just steam them and drizzle them with olive oil and lemon juice. The bottom line is, please just eat them.

Ingredients

1 leek, washed thoroughly and sliced

2 teaspoons organic coconut oil

27 oz water or vegetable stock, or water flavored with ½ teaspoon Herbamare (available in supermarkets)

1 bunch endive or chicory, chopped

1 broccoli floret, chopped

Leaves from one bunch of beets

2 medium zucchinis, chopped

Method

Heat the coconut oil gently in a large pot and add the chopped leek. Saute for 3 to 4 minutes, until softened. Add all remaining ingredients, bring to the boil and then reduce heat to a gentle simmer. Cook until all vegetables are softened. You can puree the soup in a blender or serve it chunky.

This soup can be served on its own as an entree but if having it as a meal, please add some cooked chicken or fish as a source of protein.

Raw beet salad for the gallbladder

This is a delicious salad full of healthy foods for your gallbladder. Try to eat it several times a week.

Ingredients

2 beets, peeled and grated medium fine

1 medium apple, grated coarsely

2 tablespoons fresh lemon juice

1 tablespoon apple cider vinegar

2 tablespoons extra virgin olive oil

1 tablespoon chia seeds *(put them in just before serving)*

Method

Combine grated beets and apple together in a bowl. Combine lemon juice, vinegar and oil together in a small bowl and whisk together well. Pour dressing over salad and toss well. Sprinkle chia seeds into salad and serve.

Best herbs for the gallbladder

St Mary's thistle *(Milk thistle/Silybum marianum)*

St Mary's thistle is arguably the most famous herb when it comes to improving liver health. **Please remember that your primary goal when trying to heal your gallbladder is to improve the health of your liver.**

Milk thistle stimulates bile production in the liver and in that way has a cleansing and flushing effect on the liver and the bile ducts that travel throughout your liver. For this reason, the herb is excellent for helping to prevent stone formation in the bile ducts within the liver, in people with or without a gallbladder.

St Mary's thistle also has some remarkable healing effects on the liver. It has hepatoprotective and hepatorestorative properties. That means it protects liver cells against harm caused by toxins, and it even helps to repair damaged liver cells. Liver cells are called hepatocytes, so you can understand how those terms originated.

St Mary's thistle also has lipotropic properties; that means it helps the liver to burn fat more efficiently, and especially helps to clear fat deposits within the liver. That means it is brilliant for anyone with a fatty liver. Fatty liver and gallstones often occur hand in hand, particularly in women.

The active ingredient in St Mary's thistle is called silymarin, so when you buy a St Mary's thistle supplement you should check the level of the active ingredient. According to research, an effective daily dose of silymarin is 420mg.

Turmeric (*Curcuma longa*)

You will be familiar with turmeric if you're a fan of Indian cuisine. It has an intense yellow color but comparatively little flavor. Turmeric stimulates the liver to make more bile and stimulates the gallbladder to secrete bile into the small intestine. It assists the conversion of cholesterol to bile acids, thereby helping to keep the bile fluid-like and assisting with the removal of cholesterol from the body.

Turmeric also has strong antioxidant properties and anti-inflammatory actions; that means it's effective for painful conditions such as arthritis and fibromyalgia.

Dandelion root (*Taraxacum officinalis*)

Dandelion root stimulates the gallbladder to contract and release bile into the small intestine. Therefore it has a cleansing effect on the gallbladder and improves fat digestion. That makes dandelion root excellent for anyone with nausea, indigestion or bloating after eating oily food. Dandelion leaves have a bitter flavor and are a healthy addition to salads, but the root is much more powerful. Dandelion root is found in the liver tonic Livatone.

Globe artichoke (*Cynara scolymus*)

Globe artichoke is a delicious vegetable you can include in your diet regularly, but it is also available in a more concentrated form in supplements. It stimulates the gallbladder to contract, therefore has a cleansing effect on this organ. It helps to lower cholesterol and improves symptoms of indigestion. Globe artichoke also has antioxidant effects and promotes the regeneration of liver cells. It is found in the liver tonic Livatone.

Peppermint *(Mentha piperita)*

Peppermint is excellent for relieving indigestion and nausea. It promotes the release of bile from the gallbladder into the small intestine and relaxes the sphincter of Oddi (valve that allows bile to enter the small intestine). Peppermint also reduces spasms of the bile ducts. You can drink peppermint tea with meals or after meals regularly and drink it to relieve the pain and discomfort of a gallbladder attack. You are best off buying loose leaf dried peppermint leaves from a health food store because they will be stronger than most brands of peppermint tea sold at the supermarket.

Boldo *(Peumus boldo)*

Boldo is an excellent remedy for gallstones because it increases bile production in the liver, bile secretion by the gallbladder and it even helps to relieve the pain of gallstones. Boldo has anti-inflammatory properties, therefore is great for anyone with an inflamed gallbladder (cholecystitis). Boldo has hepatoprotective properties and can help to normalize an inflamed liver. The herb is native to Chile and boldo tea is commonly consumed in most parts of South America. You can find boldo tea in South American grocery stores or delis and we strongly recommend you purchase some.

3. Keep your bowel moving and avoid constipation

Constipation is a major promoter of gallstone formation because it reduces the ability of your body to excrete excess fats, bile, cholesterol and toxins. Therefore these wastes get reabsorbed back into the body and place a strain on the liver.

It is important to have between one and three thorough bowel movements each day if you want to dissolve gallstones and heal your gallbladder

Therefore you will need to drink plenty of water, and have adequate amounts of the right fiber in your diet to achieve this. Grains are the foods most well known for their fiber content, but they are a common cause of irritable bowel syndrome and therefore you may be better off avoiding them. Grains are also a common cause of food sensitivities, and in that way can impair normal gallbladder function. This topic is covered in more detail in point six.

A normal, healthy stool is a medium brown color, and a soft log shape. It should hold together in the bowl and not fall apart. The stool should not be small, hard or difficult to pass. It should also not smell overly strong. Bile has a deodorising effect on the stool and people with gallbladder disease usually do not secrete enough bile into their intestines. Therefore they are more prone to having overly offensive smelling stools.

Constipation puts a great strain on your liver and gallbladder

After you have digested the food in your intestines and broken it down into its building blocks, most of the nutrients get absorbed into your bloodstream via a vein called the hepatic portal vein. This vein travels directly to your liver.

If you are having regular, thorough bowel movements, the waste in your intestines will be eliminated from your body. However, in a constipated person, the waste remains in the intestines for a much longer period of time, and consequently some of that waste gets reabsorbed back into the bloodstream, and travels straight to the liver.

Constipation also worsens the common hormone imbalance in women known as estrogen dominance and relative progesterone deficiency. Women are supposed to break down large quantities of estrogen each day in their liver, and excrete it in bowel motions. Constipated women reabsorb much of that estrogen and it ends up recirculating back to the liver. This can produce unpleasant symptoms such as PMS, menstrual cramps, heavy periods and tender breasts, but it can also raise the risk of breast or uterine cancer in the future.

In terms of gallstones, constipation in women is a problem because it raises estrogen levels and estrogen increases the amount of cholesterol in bile, thus leading to thicker bile that is more likely to form stones.

Strategies for overcoming constipation

Some people can easily and quickly resolve their constipation just by drinking more water and following a healthy diet. Unfortunately for others the solution is not so simple.

A great range of conditions and factors can cause constipation and sometimes fixing the problem is as difficult as solving a murder mystery. Women are more likely to suffer with constipation than men and it is more common in people over the age of 65.

Here are some methods that help most people overcome constipation. Hopefully you'll find something that works for you:

- Drink approximately eight to ten glasses of water or herbal tea each day. Coffee and tea do not count. Tea can make constipation worse because of the tannins it contains.

- Have a blood test to check if you have an underactive thyroid. This is an incredibly common cause of constipation in women. Have a blood test for the hormone called TSH (Thyroid Stimulating Hormone). Your blood level should be between 0.3 and 2.5 IU/L. For more information see our book *Your Thyroid Problems Solved*. We have found there are an enormous amount of women who fall into the gray zone, where their thyroid is not perfect but not yet bad enough for their doctor to pay attention and offer any solutions. This condition is known as subclinical hypothyroidism and it can have a very negative effect on your health and quality of life.

- Make sure you are eating a large volume of fresh vegetables each day. Some can be cooked and some should be raw. Aim for approximately 5 fists full of vegetables each day and one or two pieces of fruit.

- Find out if you have a hidden food sensitivity. This is a very common yet under appreciated cause of constipation. The most common culprits are gluten, dairy products, soy, corn, eggs and nuts. It is best to see a naturopath or nutritionist who can help you uncover which foods may be upsetting your digestion. Removal of a problematic food can produce a dramatic improvement in bowel function.

- Don't ignore the urge to have a bowel movement. It may not be the most convenient time or place, but that doesn't matter. Holding on for too long can upset healthy digestion and make you more prone to constipation in the future.

- Include fermented foods in your diet regularly. Learn how to make them at home or buy them from a health food store. Examples include sauerkraut, kimchi or kefir (which does not have to be made in milk). Coconut yogurt is another healthy food to include in your diet. You can buy it in health food stores or make it yourself.

- You might have an overgrowth of bad bacteria, yeast, fungi and Candida in your bowel. This can cause constipation, bloating, flatulence, indigestion and nausea. There are some brilliant herbal products that act as a powerful anti-microbial in the bowel. I recommend a formula containing the herbs cloves, black walnut, pau d'arco and garlic. You can find these combined in capsule form called Intestinal Parasite Cleanse capsules.

- Consider taking a probiotic (good bowel bacteria supplement). A probiotic can mean the difference between healthy bowel habits and chronic constipation. We see that regularly at our clinics.

- Make sure you are eating enough healthy fats, as good fats help to lubricate the bowel. See page 54 for our recommended healthy fats.

- Add a gentle source of fiber to your diet such as chia seeds, freshly ground flaxseeds, slippery elm or psyllium. This fiber can be added to smoothies, vegetable juices, sprinkled over salad with your lunch or sprinkled over chopped fruit and eaten as a snack. I recommend Fibertone powder, which is a combination of slippery elm, rice bran, peppermint, ginger and other beneficial ingredients for the bowel. The dose of this fiber supplement is two teaspoons twice daily. For more information you could call our health advisory line on 1888 755 4837.

- Magnesium promotes healthy bowel function because it relaxes the nerves and muscles of the bowel. In this way it is very helpful for people who hold their stress and tension in their bowel and experience constipation when stressed or travelling. A good dose of Magnesium Ultra Potent powder is 400mg per day and this can be achieved with one teaspoon of magnesium powder daily, taken with or without meals.

- Vitamin C helps relieve constipation by softening the stool. You can take as much vitamin C as you need to promote a bowel motion. Start with 4000mg of vitamin C per day and increase the dose until you achieve the desired outcome. Vitamin C has numerous benefits in the body and can be safely taken long term, but reserve very high doses to those times when you're constipated and your usual tricks aren't working.

- Some medications can promote constipation; these include some antidepressants, some analgesics, aluminium containing antacids, calcium channel blockers (used for high blood pressure) and some types of calcium and iron supplements.

- Stress management may be a critical component of addressing constipation. Meditation, yoga, deep breathing, counselling or spending more time on fun hobbies and with fun friends may be helpful.

- Exercise is important because it stimulates intestinal contractions, called peristalsis. Getting some kind of movement each day is very important, even if it's just a walk.

4. Take the right nutrients necessary for healthy bile

Healthy bile is critical for a healthy gallbladder. There are several explanations for why gallbladder disease is so common; one of them is inadequate levels of the nutrients critical for healthy bile production. If you do not get enough of these nutrients in your diet, the bile you produce may be too rich in cholesterol and too low in bile acids. That scenario encourages stone formation.

These nutrients and supplements primarily work by increasing bile acids.

Taurine and glycine

The production of bile involves the conjugation (binding) of cholesterol to one of two amino acids - glycine or taurine. These amino acids are both found in protein rich foods such as poultry, seafood, eggs and meat. Most of you probably have plenty of these amino acids in your diet, however if you suffer with poor digestion, you may not be absorbing them adequately. Also, if the amount of cholesterol in your body is relatively high, there may be inadequate levels of glycine and taurine in your body to compensate.

Taking a supplement that contains taurine and glycine can help to improve the production of healthy bile. It will also help with the removal of excess cholesterol from your body. An effective dose is between 1000 and 2000mg of taurine and glycine each day, taken with food.

Ox bile

Ox bile probably doesn't sound very appealing to you, but the difference it can make to your health is amazing.

Taking an ox bile supplement should help to improve your digestion and make you feel more comfortable after meals, but it will also help to dissolve any stones you may have in your gallbladder.

Ox bile actually comes from bovine sources (cows) and it is purified and freeze dried to maintain its potency. It is an alternative to taking the prescription medication Ursofalk (ursodeoxycholic acid), used for dissolving gallstones.

Ox bile will help to make your bile less thick and sludgy and will work on dissolving any stones you may have in your gallbladder. It helps to reduce pain and indigestion after meals and helps you digest fat more effectively. People with pale (tan colored) stools, bloating, indigestion and nausea have strong indicators of bile insufficiency. Taking an ox bile supplement is excellent for relieving these symptoms. If you suffer with dry skin and hair, you should find that ox bile helps improve those symptoms by enabling you to digest good fats more efficiently.

Ox bile must be taken with meals and a typical dose is between 100 and 500mg with each meal. Taking too much can give you loose bowel motions, so just cut down the dose. For more information on ox bile see www.liverdoctor.com

Vitamin C

You have probably never thought of vitamin C in relation to gallstones but it's needed by the enzyme that converts cholesterol into bile acids. The name of this enzyme is 7-hydroxylase. Therefore vitamin C reduces the risk of gallstone formation and helps to dissolve stones already present. Many people don't get enough vitamin C in their diet because they don't eat enough raw fresh fruit and vegetables, or the produce has lost much of its vitamin C content because it has been stored for long periods of time after harvest. Vitamin C is very fragile and easily destroyed by cooking. If you have gallstones, we recommend you supplement with four grams of vitamin C daily, taken in two 2 gram doses.

Magnesium

People with a higher intake of magnesium are less likely to experience gallstones. Magnesium helps to improve insulin sensitivity and in that way is very helpful for people with syndrome X or insulin resistance.

High blood insulin levels drive the liver to manufacture more cholesterol, and in that way promote gallstone formation. Magnesium helps to reverse that process. A study conducted in men and published in the American Journal of Gastroenterology found that men with the highest daily intake of magnesium were 28 percent less likely to develop gallstones than men with the lowest magnesium intake. [7.]

Magnesium also relaxes the muscles of the body, including the smooth muscle of the bile ducts. In this way magnesium reduces spasms and pain associated with biliary colic and a gallbladder attack. The recommended dose of magnesium is between 400 and 600mg per day and you can find a magnesium powder combined with malic acid called Magnesium Ultra Potent powder.

Selenium

Selenium is a mineral that helps to support liver function and detoxification. Selenium supplements are most effective in the selenomethionine form. Selenium helps to support healthy bile production and bile is an important route for the elimination of toxins from the liver.

N-acetyl cysteine (NAC)

The natural compound NAC supports glutathione production in the liver and therefore supports detoxification. N-acetyl cysteine reduces inflammation in the liver lobules where the tiny bile ducts originate.

Apple cider vinegar and malic acid

Apple cider vinegar is an inexpensive, effective remedy for helping to dissolve gallstones and helping to improve your digestion. Problems with digestion are commonly associated with gallstones and we have covered this topic in point number six in this chapter. Apple cider vinegar is excellent for people with low stomach acid and poor protein digestion. It helps reduce bloating, indigestion, burping and flatulence. Vinegar helps glucose metabolism; it reduces your blood sugar level after a meal. This is especially beneficial for people with diabetes or syndrome X, which are risk factors for gallstones.

The malic acid in apple cider vinegar helps to soften gallstones and make the bile more fluid and thin, and less thick and sludge-like. We recommend you add one to two tablespoons of apple cider vinegar to a quarter of a cup of warm water and sip it five minutes before each meal. If you forget to drink it before your meal, have it during the meal. It will prepare your digestive organs for the meal and help you extract more nutrients from your food. Organic apple cider vinegar is preferable.

Coffee

Regular coffee drinkers are less likely to develop gallstones than people who don't drink coffee. This is probably because coffee triggers the release of bile from the gallbladder, therefore reducing the risk of bile stasis. Research has shown that, compared to people who drink no coffee at all, men who drink two or more cups of coffee a day are 40 to 45 percent less likely to develop gallstones. [8]

In women the risk is reduced by 22 to 28 percent. [9]

Melatonin

You may have heard of melatonin as a remedy for insomnia, but surprisingly it has several properties that make it a valuable remedy for the gallbladder. Melatonin is a hormone that is secreted by the pineal gland in the brain, and also by the digestive tract. It helps to regulate your body clock and enables you to sleep during the night and be awake during the day. Melatonin is traditionally given to people with jet lag to help them recover normal sleeping patterns. Melatonin is also known to function as an antioxidant and helps to reduce the risk of cancer.

Recent research has shown melatonin can prevent and treat gallstones in several ways. Inflammation of the gallbladder walls (cholecystitis) can cause pain and it also predisposes to gallstone formation. Melatonin acts as an antioxidant and helps to protect the cells lining the inside of the gallbladder from oxidative harm.

Melatonin reduces the amount of cholesterol in bile by inhibiting reabsorption of cholesterol in the intestines, and aiding the conversion of cholesterol to bile salts. [10.]

5. Reduce cholesterol

Cholesterol on the whole is very good for you; it performs many vital functions in your body. You just don't want too much of it in your bile. The most common type of gallstones are the ones made from cholesterol. When there is too much cholesterol in your bile, we refer to the condition as cholesterol super-saturation. So essentially there is too much cholesterol relative to the bile acids within the bile, and that promotes biliary sludge and eventually stones.

Having a high level of cholesterol in your blood is not always a bad thing and it must be taken in context with other health status indicators such as blood pressure, triglycerides, blood sugar and others. If you have high blood cholesterol and you also have a gallbladder problem, chances are you probably eat too much carbohydrate and you have syndrome X.

Syndrome X is also known as insulin resistance or metabolic syndrome. People with syndrome X have higher blood insulin levels than ideal, and the insulin is becoming less and less effective at regulating the blood sugar level. Syndrome X causes abdominal weight gain and raises your risk of developing type 2 diabetes.

Syndrome X is diagnosed using the following criteria:

- Fasting blood glucose equal to or greater than 99 mg/dL.
- Blood pressure equal to or higher than 130/85 mmHg.
- Waist circumference greater than 31 inches in women and 37 inches in men.
- Triglycerides (blood fats) equal to or greater than 168 mg/dL.
- HDL (good) cholesterol less than 50 mg/dL in women and less than 40 mg/dL in men.

The most effective way to keep your cholesterol in the healthy range is to keep your blood insulin level low. This is because insulin is the signal that prompts your liver to manufacture cholesterol. The more cholesterol your liver makes, the more will eventually end up in your bile, aggravating your gallbladder problem.

Which foods raise cholesterol?

You will not get high cholesterol from eating saturated fat or cholesterol. Carbohydrate rich foods, as well as some processed, omega 6 rich vegetable oils are the big culprits in raising your cholesterol. Therefore they are the foods you must get rid of from your diet, or significantly reduce your consumption of.

The following foods raise cholesterol and should be avoided:

- Sugar
- Sweet drinks - soda drinks, sports drinks, fruit juice, cordial
- Foods made of flour - bread, pasta, cakes, cookies, crackers, wraps
- Salty carbohydrates - potato chips, corn chips, pretzels
- Alcohol
- Breakfast cereals
- Polenta, cous cous, semolina, pasta, noodles
- Grains - rice, corn, wheat and others.

You do not have to remove every last trace of these foods from your diet, but you will need to at least significantly cut down. Clearly you developed gallstones for a reason, so you need to change the metabolism of your body so it no longer promotes gallstone formation.

So what can I eat?

You will need to base your diet on vegetables, salads, seafood, poultry, eggs, meat (preferably grass fed/pasture raised), along with good fats. Suitable sources of good fats include extra virgin olive oil, avocados, coconut oil, macadamia nut oil and avocado oil. Small quantities of raw nuts and seeds are fine as long as they don't give you digestive problems.

The average person's diet is quite high in carbohydrate, so it may be quite a shock to the system to try and reduce these foods in your diet.

Carbohydrate rich foods are convenient, tasty and crave worthy. Unfortunately excess amounts of dietary carbohydrates spell trouble for your liver and gallbladder.

Whenever you eat carbohydrate rich food, such as bread, pasta, potatoes, rice or biscuits, they are broken down and digested by you into their building block - glucose. It really doesn't matter whether the carbohydrate rich food has a high or low glycaemic index; in the end it becomes glucose. Therefore, eating these foods produces a rise in your blood glucose level.

When your blood glucose rises, your pancreas senses this and releases insulin into your blood. Insulin tells your liver to store some of the glucose inside it, in the form glycogen, and some gets stored in your muscles. Unfortunately your body only has a small amount of storage space for glycogen (there is even less room in your liver if you have a fatty liver). Once there is no more room to store glucose as glycogen, your liver converts the excess glucose into fat instead.

Therefore insulin is released into your bloodstream each time you eat carbohydrate, and insulin stimulates your liver to produce fat and store it. Some fat gets stored within your liver and some gets deposited around your body as general fat stores. Some triglycerides get repackaged into cholesterol molecules, and some of this cholesterol will end up in your bile inside your gallbladder. If the cholesterol level in your bile reaches super-saturation point, that is a recipe for gallstone formation.

Several studies have shown that the more sugar a person eats, the greater their risk of developing gallstones [11]

Fructose is the sugar found in fruit and also table sugar (sucrose), which is composed of a glucose molecule bound to a fructose molecule. Fructose is particularly problematic because it cannot be used by your cells directly for energy; it must be taken to the liver to be used for energy. The human body preferably converts fructose into fat.[12.] This means fructose can raise your blood fats more significantly than glucose. Therefore anyone wishing to lose weight, lower their cholesterol or dissolve gallstones should limit their fruit intake to not more than two servings per day.

Inflammation raises cholesterol too

Recent research has found that the more inflammation is present in your body, the greater your cholesterol level tends to be. Inflammation is a bit of a vague term that you've probably seen mentioned recently. There are two main types of inflammation: acute inflammation and chronic inflammation.

If you have ever sprained your ankle or suffered a gout attack, you'll know all about acute inflammation. It causes symptoms like pain, swelling, heat, redness and immobility.

Chronic inflammation is quite different. This is the type of inflammation that occurs in a very subtle form inside your body, so you don't even realize it's occurring.

Chronic inflammation occurs when various cells in your body produce chemicals that cause wear and tear inside your body. Essentially, inflammation causes oxidative damage to the cells and tissues of your body. This will cause you to age more rapidly and put you at risk of serious diseases including cardiovascular disease and cancer. Inflammatory chemicals can be produced by your immune cells, fat cells and by your liver if it is fatty, otherwise diseased or sluggish.

What causes inflammation and how is it relevant to cholesterol?

The following factors all raise the level of inflammation in your body:

- Being overweight
- Diabetes
- Infections
- Stress

- Lack of sleep
- Deficiency of omega 3 fats in the diet
- Lack of fresh vegetables in the diet
- Food allergy or intolerance
- Diets high in sugar, alcohol, gluten and omega 6 fats
- Nutritional deficiencies, especially of vitamin C, vitamin D and selenium

In most people, the overwhelming cause of excessive inflammation in their body is poor dietary choices. Sugar, flour and vegetable oil high in omega 6 fats (soy, corn, cottonseed, sunflower, safflower oil) all cause wear and tear to your body. Having a fatty liver causes the liver to produce high levels of damaging inflammatory chemicals.

Cholesterol has a vital role in healing and repair of tissues in your body. Therefore if the level of inflammation is high, the need for tissue repair is also high. The problem is, too much cholesterol in your body can start to have harmful consequences for your arteries and for your gallbladder. If you concentrate on lowering the inflammation in your body, you should be able to also lower your cholesterol.

6. Avoid problem foods and fix your digestion

The old fashioned advice given to gallbladder patients was to just eat less fat. Don't eat greasy or oily meals and that way you won't develop a gallbladder problem in the first place, or if you have one already, you can cure it with a low fat diet. This is unhelpful advice and really doesn't work for most people with a gallbladder problem.

Most people with an inflamed gallbladder or gallstones will find there are specific foods that cause great pain and discomfort. We refer to these foods as trigger foods because they can trigger discomfort in someone with a disgruntled gallbladder, but they can also trigger an acute gallbladder attack in a person with more advanced gallbladder disease. If you are regularly in discomfort and want to avoid an emergency hospital trip, these are the foods you must steer clear of.

Digestive problems

Digestive problems are commonly associated with gallstones. Some people are not surprised to discover they have gallstones because they have wined and dined and eaten their way through a parade of rich foods and sugary treats. However, sometimes people who are very careful with their diet and who try to eat healthy foods still develop gallstones. Sometimes the gallstones develop very early in life, such as the early 20s. These are the atypical gallbladder patients and we have to suspect that something is very wrong with their digestion and liver function.

Food intolerance, irritable bowel syndrome, celiac disease, pancreatic insufficiency and insufficient stomach acid (hypochlorhydria) can all increase the risk of gallstones. Digestive problems can increase the risk of gallbladder disease by interfering with the ability of the gallbladder to contract properly.

Celiac disease and gallstones

Celiac disease is a severe form of gluten intolerance whereby ingesting gluten prompts an autoimmune reaction in the body. Gluten is found in wheat, rye, barley, spelt, triticale, oats, kamut and many processed foods that contain any of these grains.

People with celiac disease develop inflammation in their intestines when they eat gluten. The hormone that stimulates the gallbladder to contract is mostly made in the first part of the small intestine called the duodenum. This hormone is called cholecystokinin (CCK) and people with celiac disease usually do not produce adequate levels if they are consuming gluten. The gluten itself also seems to interfere with the ability of the gallbladder to contract because celiacs commonly have a very low bile ejection fraction during a HIDA scan if they are regularly consuming gluten.

A small study comparing the ability of the gallbladder to contract recruited six healthy volunteers, six people with untreated celiac disease (they were eating gluten) and six people with treated celiac disease (they were following a gluten free diet). All study subjects were asked to drink a liquid fatty meal in the morning, following an overnight fast. The researchers measured the average time it took for their gallbladder to empty by 50 percent.

In the healthy people and the celiacs on a gluten free diet it took an average of 20 minutes for their gallbladder to empty by half. It was a very different story in the untreated celiacs; it took their gallbladder an average of 154 minutes to empty by half. The authors of the study concluded that celiac disease can cause a gallbladder emptying defect that is reversible with a gluten free diet. [13.]

Sometimes gallstones are the first manifestation of celiac disease in people who weren't aware they have the condition. They typically occur early in life, in the 20s or early 30s. Celiacs are also more likely to suffer with atresia, which is a partial or complete blockage of a bile duct.

Unfortunately people with celiac disease or any other food sensitivity are the ones most likely to still experience pain and discomfort after having their gallbladder removed. This is simply because there was nothing wrong with the gallbladder itself; it was just not able to function correctly while the patient was eating foods that don't agree with them. It is a tragedy when these food sensitivities aren't discovered until after the patient has lost an important organ.

Food allergies and gallstones

There are several terms used to describe an adverse reaction to a food - food allergy, food intolerance or food sensitivity. These different reactions to foods can affect different branches of the immune system and vary greatly in the types of reactions they can produce. For our purposes, we will refer to all the various adverse reactions to foods as food sensitivities.

If you regularly eat a food your body cannot digest properly, or that your immune system considers a threat, you will mount an inflammatory response to that food

Food sensitivities can cause wide ranging, unexpected reactions in virtually any organ or tissue of the body. They can behave unpredictably and that makes identifying the problem very tricky. Anyone with a food sensitivity will experience some inflammation in their digestive tract, and this irritates the immune cells that live in the intestines.

If you eat a food that your digestive system cannot properly break down, the remnants will provide food for unhealthy bacteria, yeast, fungi and Candida in your digestive tract. That further aggravates your health and contributes to other symptoms.

Everyone with food sensitivities would greatly benefit from a glutamine supplement. Glutamine is an amino acid which helps to soothe and repair an irritated or inflamed digestive lining. It is actually used as fuel by the cells that line the digestive tract. An effective dose of glutamine is two grams of powder twice daily taken away from food. An inflamed small intestine interferes with proper release of the hormone cholecystokinin, therefore interferes with proper gallbladder contraction.

It is interesting to see that research has been done on food sensitivities and gallbladder disease. A study performed on 69 patients showed that the avoidance of allergenic foods eliminated gallbladder symptoms in one hundred percent of patients with gallstones or post-cholecystectomy syndrome (pain and symptoms after gallbladder removal). The patients were aged between 31 and 97 years and they were placed on an elimination diet, eating only a handful of foods for one week. Interestingly their fat intake was not restricted.

After following the elimination diet for a week, one food was introduced at a time to watch for a reaction. Remarkably, while on the elimination diet, every single one of the 69 patients was symptom free. Improvements took three to five days to appear. Eggs, pork and onions were the most common problematic foods, with reaction by 93, 64 and 52 percent of people respectively. [14.]

The table below lists the problematic foods and percentage of patients who reacted to them. You can use it as a guide to determine which foods affect your gallbladder.

Offending food	Percentage of patients reacting
eggs	93
pork	64
onions	52
chicken	35
milk	25
coffee	22
oranges	19
corn	15
beans (legumes)	15
nuts	15
apples	6
tomatoes	6

This particular study didn't include gluten, which other research, and our own experience has shown to be very problematic for the gallbladder.

The author of this study wisely stated that the standard dietary recommendations to avoid fatty, greasy and rich foods may not be the best advice for patients with gallbladder disease. The name of the study is *Allergy elimination diet as the most effective gallbladder diet* and it was published way back in 1968. Why is it that such a brilliant study has been largely forgotten, and the average doctor is still telling their patients with gallbladder disease to eat less fat?

An elimination diet works best for people with early stage gallbladder disease or people with not many gallstones, or none at all but lots of symptoms. When the gallbladder has been unhealthy for years, there are several stones and the walls have thickened, it takes much longer to experience an improvement.

Worst foods for the gallbladder

According to that list above, and our patient experience, the worst foods for the gallbladder are gluten, sugar, eggs, pork, onions and dairy products. Therefore we strongly recommend you avoid those foods while trying to heal your gallbladder, and avoid all junk food as well.

We consider onions, eggs and free range pork to be healthy foods that the average person can safely include in their diet; however if you have gallbladder disease, you are best off to stay away from them for now.

Dairy products are not recommended for anyone with a liver, intestinal or gallbladder condition. They can promote a gallbladder attack, can inflame the gallbladder and promote the growth of gallstones. Here are the reasons why dairy products are so problematic:

- Dairy products are one of the most common foods people have an allergy or intolerance to. Food allergy or intolerance can interfere with the ability of your gallbladder to contract properly, thus promoting stasis of bile. It is the protein in dairy products that promotes food intolerance. The protein is called casein. That means lactose free milk is not suitable because it still contains casein.

- Some dairy products are high in fat and dairy fat is notorious for triggering a gallbladder attack. Having said that, skim milk isn't suitable because it still contains casein.

- Dairy products are mucus forming foods and they tend to thicken the body's secretions, from the sinuses, throat, lungs and digestive tract. People who eat dairy products may have thicker bile and thick bile is more likely to form sludge and eventual stones.

A2 milk is significantly less likely to promote a food allergy or intolerance but we do not recommend this type of milk either if you are wishing to resolve your gallbladder problem. If you must drink milk, coconut milk, almond milk and hemp milk are best. You could make your own milk out of any nut or seed, using a powerful blender. There are numerous instructional videos on YouTube.

Low stomach acid and gallbladder disease

Low stomach acid is also known as hypochlorhydria and it is very common in people with gallbladder disease and food allergies. In one study, 52 percent of patients with gallstones were found to have low stomach acid. [15.]

Symptoms of low stomach acid are typical in people with gallbladder disease; they include burping, flatulence, abdominal bloating, abdominal pain and nausea. Low stomach acid favors the growth of bad bacteria in the stomach and intestines, leading to dysbiosis, which means an unfavorable balance of bugs in the digestive tract.

You can take a supplement of hydrochloric acid, which is called betaine hydrochloride. Low stomach acid usually occurs hand in hand with low levels of digestive enzymes. Taking a good digestive enzyme supplement such as Super Digestive Enzymes will help to relieve the symptoms of indigestion and will help you absorb more nutrients from your meals and supplements. The Super Digestive Enzymes supplement contains betaine hydrochloride, ox bile and pancreatic enzymes all in one capsule. For more information see www.liverdoctor.com. Sipping apple cider vinegar before meals also supports stomach acid production.

Identifying and eliminating food allergies will help to raise your own body's production of digestive enzymes and hydrochloric acid in time. Stress and anxiety are another common cause of low stomach acid and digestive enzymes. You can increase your own body's production of hydrochloric acid by eating the bitter foods and herbs listed in point two in this chapter.

Foods to avoid and foods to include in your diet if you want to heal your gallbladder

Through our clinical experience, these are the foods we have seen most commonly trigger a gallbladder attack or gallbladder pain. The list may be slightly different in your case or there may be additional foods that make you feel unwell. Therefore please avoid any food that you know or suspect upsets you. Use our list as a guideline but please listen to your body; it will tell you which foods aren't appropriate for you if you listen carefully.

Good foods	Bad foods
Eat more	*Eat less or avoid altogether*
Beet leaves	Dairy products - eg. milk, cheese, yogurt
Beets	
Chicory	Gluten - wheat, rye, oats, barley, spelt
Endive	Sugar
Dandelion leaves	Eggs
Globe artichoke	Onions
Radishes - red and daikon	Pork
Lemons and limes	Polyunsaturated vegetable oil derived from most seeds and nuts
Turmeric - fresh rhizome or dried and ground	
All vegetables - except potatoes	Margarine and non-dairy spread
All fruit but limit to two serves a day	Gluten free foods (bread, pasta, etc.) should be avoided or kept to a minimum
Fish and other seafood	
Poultry	
Red meat	
- preferably grass fed	
Good fats - avocados, olive, macadamia, avocado or coconut oil	
Fresh herbs (arugula, basil, watercress)	
Cabbage	
Kale	

Nuts, seeds and legumes can be eaten in small quantities if you feel you can digest them well. If you suffer with irritable bowel syndrome or several food allergies, it is best to avoid these foods for now while your digestive system is healing. Some people are able to digest nuts better if they have been soaked beforehand or ground in a food processor or coffee grinder.

Sample meal plan:

A day in the life of someone trying to heal their gallbladder

This sample meal plan is for ideas only. You do not have to follow it precisely in order to get good results.

At the beginning of breakfast

A quarter of a cup of warm water with a tablespoon of apple cider vinegar.

Breakfast

Protein powder smoothie made of pea, hemp or rice protein, blended with water, raw fruit, coconut oil and chia seeds.
or
Left overs from dinner such as chicken soup or salmon with salad
or
Quinoa porridge made with diluted coconut milk or almond milk

At the beginning of lunch

A quarter of a cup of warm water with a tablespoon of apple cider vinegar.

Lunch

Canned salmon, tuna, mackerel or sardines with salad, dressed with lemon juice and olive oil
or
Grilled chicken salad dressed with lemon juice and olive oil
or
Lamb curry, made with lots of vegetables and served without rice, noodles or bread

At the beginning of dinner

A quarter of a cup of warm water with a tablespoon of apple cider vinegar.

Dinner

Beef stir fry with plenty of vegetables but without noodles or rice
or
Roast chicken or baked fish with roasted vegetables or salad
or
Green soup for the gallbladder (recipe in chapter twelve) served with baked fish

You can drink a glass of raw vegetable juice (recipe in chapter twelve) once or twice each day, whenever it's most convenient for you.

Snacks and dessert

If you feel hungry, you can eat fresh fruit or raw vegetable sticks dipped in hummus, tahini or mashed avocado.

7. Eat the right fats.

Fat can be very good or very bad for the gallbladder; it all depends on the type of fat you eat and the quantity. We certainly do not recommend a low fat diet for anyone with gallbladder disease, as we explained in our first point. However it's also critical to avoid big meals containing a lot of fat.

When food enters your small intestine, it triggers release of the hormone cholecystokinin (CCK) from the intestinal cells. This hormone stimulates contractions of the gallbladder. Fat, more than any other nutrient stimulates the release of CCK. Therefore the more fat you eat, the more powerful the gallbladder contractions become.

If you regularly experience mild to moderate discomfort in your gallbladder after most meals, you are at serious risk of a severe gallbladder attack if you eat a huge meal that has too much fat in it

Bad fats for the gallbladder

- Margarine and all dairy free spreads
- Vegetable oils high in omega 6 fats and damaged fats including cottonseed oil, canola, sunflower, safflower, corn, soybean, grapeseed and rice bran oil.
- Foods cooked with vegetable oil/fat, such as cookies, crackers, takeaway food, hot chips.
- Processed foods containing vegetable oil, such as salad dressings, mayonnaise, pesto, sundried tomatoes, sauces, soy milk and any other food where you see the words "vegetable oil" on the label.
- Fat found in dairy products such as butter, cream and cheese. Fat free versions of these foods are not suitable either. Anyone wishing to heal their gallbladder should avoid all dairy products.
- Deep fried foods such as fries, donuts or chicken nuggets.

Margarine and most vegetable oils are very high in omega 6 fats. Fatty acids are fragile molecules, and these fats are particularly delicate and prone to oxidation (damage). Most vegetable oils are extracted from seeds using high heat, pressure and chemical solvents. The manufacturing process damages the fatty acids and forms what is known as products of lipid peroxidation. These molecules are highly inflammatory and create free radical damage throughout the body. They are implicated as a causative factor in cancer, heart disease, depression, infertility, accelerated aging, and any condition where pain is a feature. These fats promote inflammation of the gallbladder and they raise cholesterol.

Some vegetable oil and margarine contain trans fats (trans fatty acids), which are even more harmful and interfere with normal cell function. Levels of trans fats in foods have been greatly reduced recently due to increasing consumer awareness of their harmful effects, but they are still present in many processed foods. If you look at the nutrition information panel of a packet of potato chips for instance, you may see a low level of trans fats of approximately 0.1 gram per 100 grams.

That isn't much, but problems occur if the food you eat for each meal and snack contains trans fats. They quickly accumulate.

Good fats for the gallbladder

- Cold pressed extra virgin olive oil

- Cold pressed macadamia nut oil.

- Cold pressed avocado oil.

- Cold pressed organic coconut oil. The fats in coconut oil are predominantly medium chain triglycerides and these fats do not require bile for their digestion. They go straight to the liver where they are used for energy. Therefore coconut oil does not place a strain on your gallbladder. However, don't go overboard with this fat; all fats should be used in moderate quantities while you are trying to heal your gallbladder.

- Avocados

- Raw nuts and seeds. That means they are not roasted and not salted. Suitable varieties include almonds, walnuts, pecans, pine nuts, Brazil nuts, cashews, hazelnuts, sunflower seeds, pumpkin seeds, chia seeds, flaxseeds and hemp seeds. Some people find nuts and seeds difficult to digest and they can be irritating to the digestive lining. If that applies to you, you may need to avoid them for the time being, or soak them before consumption.

- Hummus, tahini and fresh nut spreads, such as the Artisana brand.

- Omega 3 fats found in fish oil, krill oil and marine algae. These fats are called EPA (Eicosahexaonoic acid) and DHA (Docosahexaenoic acid). They are strongly anti-inflammatory and are greatly lacking in the average person's diet. These fats help to repair damaged cell membranes and they help to keep blood cholesterol and triglyceride levels within a healthy range.

Oily fish such as sardines, salmon, mackerel, herrings, trout and anchovies are all good sources of these fats if they are wild (not farmed). However, to ensure optimum intake, it is best to take these oils in supplement form, along with a supplement containing digestive enzymes and ox bile, to ensure you digest them properly. The optimum dose in supplement form is approximately 1.2 grams of EPA and 800 mg of DHA each day, with meals. That usually equates to 4 capsules per day of a high strength fish oil product. Take two capsules twice daily and have them just before food. Krill oil is much lower in EPA and DHA than fish oil, so you would need to take quite a lot of capsules per day to achieve that dose. Studies have shown that people who consume more oily fish are less likely to develop gallstones [16] and fish oil helps to keep the cholesterol in bile soluble, thus making it less likely that stones will develop. [17]

- Small quantities of ghee, lard and tallow are suitable for cooking, because they are heat stable and do not promote inflammation. Through trial and error you can determine if these fats suit you and your gallbladder or not. Coconut oil is also suitable for cooking because it does not get damaged (oxidized) by heat.

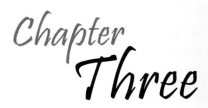

Chapter
Three

First aid remedies for easing the pain of a gallbladder attack

Here are some remedies you can easily perform at home to ease your pain and shorten the duration of a gallbladder attack. These remedies should work for a mild to moderate gallbladder attack, but if you are in severe pain, or the attack lasts longer than four hours, please go to a hospital.

Simple hot pack

The purpose of applying heat to your gallbladder is to expand the bile ducts and relieve pressure. This can be very effective for calming down painful spasms of the biliary ducts, and if a small stone is trapped in a bile duct, the application of heat may relieve the blockage.

You will need a warm moist towel and either a hot water bottle or a heated wheat bag. Lie down and place a warm moist towel on the upper part of the right side of your abdomen. Apply a hot water bottle on top of the towel and leave it in place for ten to 15 minutes.

After that time, get up, walk around for a couple of minutes and then lie down again and repeat the procedure. You can repeat this process several times until the gallbladder attack passes.

Castor oil hot pack

A castor oil hot pack is more effective than using a hot water bottle or wheat bag.

Castor oil comes from the seed of the castor bean plant called Ricinus communis. Castor oil is commonly used in a heat pack or compress to treat a variety of painful conditions, including menstrual pain and joint pain.

When it comes to gallbladder attacks, castor oil can relieve pain and spasms of the gallbladder and bile ducts. The castor oil also gets absorbed through your skin and has healing properties. Therefore it is beneficial to apply a castor oil hot pack to your gallbladder and liver during an acute gallbladder attack, but we also suggest you use this remedy regularly, for 30 minutes, three times a week at least two hours after dinner if you have an inflamed gallbladder that regularly causes you discomfort.

A word of warning; castor oil has quite a strong offensive odor and it can leave permanent stains on your clothing, bed sheets, towels, etcetera. So make sure you use old towels and sheets that you don't mind ruining.

Directions for making a castor oil pack

You will need the following equipment:
- castor oil (cold pressed is best)
- plastic cling wrap
- one old bath towel that is warm and moist
- a cotton tea towel
- two old blankets
- a hot water bottle, half filled with hot, not boiling water

You will need to lie down in bed for half an hour with the hot pack over your gallbladder. To avoid making your bed dirty from castor oil, put an old blanket down on the spot you plan to lie on.

Soak the tea towel in castor oil. Wring the excess oil out of it and fold it in half. Lie on your back. You can place a pillow under your knees if you find that more comfortable. Place the oil stained tea towel that has been folded in half over your gallbladder area. Place a layer of cling wrap over the tea towel and put the warm, moist towel that has been folded in half over that. Place the hot water bottle on top and then the other old blanket over it. Lie there, breathing slowly and deeply for 30 minutes.

Once you have finished, remove all the layers and place the towels and blankets together in the washing machine, washing them separately from any other laundry. This entire process is cumbersome and smelly, but it can offer immense pain relief.

If you become excessively hot and uncomfortable during the process, it is fine to remove the hot water bottle for a period of time, until you feel comfortable again.

Beverages that offer relief for gallbladder pain

Flaxseed (linseed) warm drink

This is an old folk remedy used by many European cultures for relieving pain and inflammation. It is excellent for spasm and inflammation of the gallbladder and biliary ducts.

Place 2 tablespoons of flaxseeds into a small pot containing 3 cups of water. Simmer the mixture on a very low heat for 20 minutes and then strain it into a mug, so you have approximately one cup of liquid. Discard the seeds. Allow the mixture to cool slightly and then sip it slowly while still warm.

Warm apple cider vinegar drink

This is excellent for relieving nausea. It is important to include apple cider vinegar in your diet regularly if you want to dissolve gallstones, but sipping on diluted apple cider vinegar during a gallbladder attack is a useful first aid remedy.

Dissolve 2 tablespoons of apple cider vinegar in one mug of warm water and sip slowly during a gallbladder attack.

Drinking **strong peppermint tea**, or **the juice of half a lemon** in a mug of warm water are also effective remedies for a gallbladder attack, or gallbladder discomfort following a meal.

You can alternate these three drinks during a gallbladder attack, or stick to the one that offers you most relief.

Magnesium helps to reduce painful gallbladder spasms, therefore dissolving half a teaspoon of Magnesium Ultra Potent powder in a little warm water should also help reduce pain. You may need to take this every 4 hours.

Chapter Four

To flush or not to flush: when is it safe and appropriate to do a gallbladder flush?

We are fairly certain that you have heard of a gallbladder flush. You may have read quite a bit about them and contemplated doing one yourself. There is quite a lot of confusing and conflicting information about gallbladder flushes on the internet. Please keep reading, so you can become aware of the facts and decide whether you'd like to follow this procedure.

A gallbladder flush is a procedure whereby a person drinks a large quantity of olive oil and lemon juice, which causes powerful contractions of the gallbladder, hopefully expelling any stones within it in the process. Sometimes a laxative such as senna or epsom salts are also taken, in order to facilitate a thorough bowel motion.

The purpose of drinking oil is to trigger gallbladder contractions. You may remember that the hormone cholecystokinin (CCK) gets released by intestinal cells each time we eat fat. If you drink half a cup of olive oil as part of a flush, you can bet your gallbladder will perform some extremely powerful contractions.

Sometimes before doing a flush, you are advised to drink apple juice for a day or two beforehand. This is because the malic acid in the apple juice helps to soften stones. Drinking lemon juice along with olive oil during the flush is said to help soften stones too. The lemon juice also plays an important role in reducing the nausea you are likely to experience after drinking a large quantity of olive oil.

Important points to consider

- If you regularly experience pain or discomfort after a meal, or you've even had some gallbladder attacks in the past, is it really sensible to drink such a huge volume of oil? The oil will force your gallbladder to contract so strongly that you will be in significantly more pain during the procedure which may even land you in hospital.

- How big are your gallstones? Will forcing them out of your gallbladder cause them to become stuck in your bile duct and create a medical emergency that ends with you having your gallbladder removed in hospital? If you turn up at the emergency department of a hospital in that state, you probably won't be getting laparoscopic (keyhole) surgery. You would be more likely to have the old fashioned open cholecystectomy which is a more risky operation with a longer recovery time.

- Does a gallbladder flush do anything about the reason you developed stones in the first place? Does it help to prevent you developing new stones? The answers are no.

- Are the things that end up in your stool even stones, or are they solid structures formed from the interaction of oil, acid, digestive enzymes and bilirubin in your intestines?

When NOT to perform a gallbladder flush

The greatest allure of the gallbladder flush is people see it as a quick fix for ridding their gallbladder of stones, hopefully ending their gallbladder problems. Unfortunately it is not that simple.

A gallbladder flush makes your gallbladder squeeze much harder than normal

If you have an inflamed gallbladder (cholecystitis), the squeezing is going to hurt.

Likewise if your bile ducts are inflamed, the gallbladder flush will also make them hurt. If there are stones in your gallbladder, stones are hard and sharp, therefore powerful contractions will hurt a lot.

If you are regularly in pain or discomfort, doing a gallbladder flush will likely greatly worsen the pain and may leave you in pain for several hours or the entire day. Worst case scenario, you could end up in hospital due to the pain.

If you have stones in your gallbladder, you need to know how big they are

There is a risk that the flush will cause a stone to get stuck in your bile duct. If that happens, the lodged stone can block the flow of bile from your liver and gallbladder, causing the bile to back up behind the stone. This puts enormous pressure on your bile ducts, which are probably already inflamed. This could lead to an infection in your bile ducts or jaundice.

How big are your stones? How wide are your bile ducts?

These are very important facts to know. The average width of the common bile duct is around 3.4 millimetres.[18] However there is a lot of individual variation and it depends on your age and the health of your liver and gallbladder.

Older people usually have a wider common bile duct. In young people 20 years old or less, the average width is 2.8 millimetres. In people aged 71 years or older, the average width is 4.1 milimetres.

An ultrasound report of your gallbladder and liver will usually provide the measurement of your own common bile duct.

Having gallstones usually makes your bile ducts expand over time, due to the extra pressure within the gallbladder and thicker bile, which places strain on the bile ducts.

Several liver diseases can cause expansion of the bile ducts due to the increased pressure within the liver.

However, everyone's bile ducts have the ability to expand to between 10 millimetres and 15 millimetres (1.0 to 1.5 centimeters) if they have to. That means, in theory if your stones are 15 millimetres (1.5 centimeters) or smaller, you can probably pass them safely out of your gallbladder, through the common bile duct and into your small intestine.

If your stones are larger than 4 centimeters, they are too big to even leave your gallbladder. That means they are not at risk of getting stuck, but also that a gallbladder flush will not be useful. The danger zone is if your stones are between 1.5 centimeters and 4.0 centimeters. These are the stones most likely to become trapped and land a person in hospital, with the end result being the loss of their gallbladder.

Large gallstones (greater than 4 centimeters) take much longer to treat because they have a very small surface area compared to their volume. That means the amount of surface area of the stone that gets exposed to herbs, nutrients and bile acids is much smaller than in stones that aren't so big.

Because they take up so much space, large stones also interfere with the ability of the gallbladder to contract efficiently, thus reducing the ability of the gallbladder to cleanse itself properly. Therefore each time the gallbladder contracts, too much bile gets left behind and is likely to thicken and lead to bile sludge. Therefore it usually takes several years for stones of that size to dissolve. Calcified stones also take much longer to dissolve.

When it is probably safe to perform a gallbladder flush

Please do not do a gallbladder flush if you currently experience pain in your gallbladder region, which is the right upper part of your abdomen.

Basically if you are symptomatic, a gallbladder flush will likely greatly worsen your symptoms and can result in a medical emergency. Therefore the only safe time to do a gallbladder flush is if you are not in regular pain or discomfort, and your stones have been confirmed as smaller than 1.5 centimeters.

If you want to perform a gallbladder flush, we suggest you follow our diet and supplement recommendations in chapter two for a minimum of six months first.

Then, and only if you are not in pain, you can probably perform a gallbladder flush if you want to.

Our recommendations in chapter two will help reduce inflammation in your gallbladder, help to thin the bile and soften the stones. A gallbladder flush would then have a greater benefit.

Please bear in mind that you don't have to do a gallbladder flush at all. It is an entirely optional component of our recommendations. You will get the best results in terms of dissolving stones and healing your gallbladder if you follow our recommendations in chapter two and stick to them long term.

Safe and effective gallbladder flush

Before reading any further, please make sure you have read this entire chapter, and ideally the whole book. A gallbladder flush is not for everyone. There are risks and dangers involved.

If you would like to perform a gallbladder flush, please follow the steps outlined here:

Day 1 through day 5

You need to drink 3 glasses of freshly squeezed juice each day. You need to make the juice yourself in a juice extractor. Store bought juice is only acceptable if you purchase it from a juice bar where it is freshly made in front of you. Juice sold in the fridge in supermarkets is not suitable. V8 juice is not suitable.

Drink 2 glasses of freshly made apple juice on an empty stomach first thing in the morning. Add one teaspoon of organic apple cider vinegar into each glass. Later that day, in the afternoon drink one glass of vegetable juice for the gallbladder; see the recipe that follows.

Please do not drink apple juice regularly. It is an important component of the preparation for a gallbladder flush, but it should not be consumed regularly because of its high sugar content. However, you can and should drink the vegetable juice described below as often as possible.

Take one teaspoon twice daily of a powder containing a combination of magnesium and malic acid. A suitable supplement is Magnesium Ultra Potent powder which contains different salts of magnesium, malic acid, taurine and selenium.

Malic acid will help to soften the stones. Malic acid is found in apples and apple cider vinegar, but you can buy it in concentrated form in a supplement.

Magnesium helps to relax the muscles in your body, including the smooth muscle lining your bile ducts. This will help to reduce painful spasms in the bile ducts during a gallbladder flush. Magnesium also has a gentle laxative effect, helping you to achieve more thorough bowel movements.

It is beneficial to take one teaspoon of magnesium and malic acid powder each day if you have a gallbladder problem, but take two teaspoons per day while preparing for the gallbladder flush

Take the magnesium and malic acid with meals.

Most people lead very busy lives, so you can make the apple juice and vegetable juice in a large batch in advance and freeze it straight after making it. Freeze it in glass jars with a lid.

Recipe for gallbladder vegetable juice

This juice is an important component of the preparation for a gallbladder flush, but we recommend you drink this juice regularly if you have a gallbladder problem, as it has an excellent cleansing and flushing effect on both the liver and gallbladder.

Ingredients   1 large beet

8 large beet leaves

8 chicory or endive leaves

2 stalks celery

¼ red onion

1 large carrot

2 red radishes

1 small apple

Method   Pass all ingredients through a juice extractor and drink.

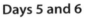

Days 5 and 6

On the evening of day 5, mix a tablespoon of epsom salts and a tablespoon of fresh lemon juice into a glass of warm water. Ideally you should drink this around half an hour before dinner. Choose a light dinner with plenty of vegetables. Two hours after dinner, have another glass of the epsom salt and lemon juice mixture.

You will need to stay home all of day 6. You will not eat any food this day. When you wake up, have another glass of epsom salts and lemon juice in warm water. Two hours later, mix half a cup of freshly squeezed lemon juice with half a cup of extra virgin olive oil. Whisk it together until it is well combined and then drink it slowly.

You will have between 4 and 10 bowel movements this day, so rest as much as possible and don't plan anything else for this weekend. If you feel very hungry in the evening of day 6, it is fine to have some cooked or raw vegetables and fruit. You can resume normal meals on day 7.

It is best to schedule day one on a Monday, so that day 6 is a Saturday and you can recover at home on Sunday (day 7) before having to go back to work.

Are you sure they were gallstones?

As far as we know, no scientific studies have been carried out whereby a large number of patients received a gallbladder ultrasound before and after a gallbladder flush to demonstrate removal of the stones via a flush. However there was a study published in the medical journal The Lancet called *Could these be gallstones?* [19.]

Researchers analysed the small stone-like objects that a 40 year old woman passed after completing a gallbladder flush where she drank an olive oil and lemon juice mixture. She collected the stones, stored them in the freezer and then delivered them to a clinic for analysis.

The stones were found to not have a crystalline structure and they melted into a green liquid when kept at 104 degrees Farenheit (40 degrees Celsius) for ten minutes. The stones were also found to not contain any cholesterol, bilirubin or calcium (normal components of gallstones).

The researchers tried to create their own stones by mixing oleic acid (the main component of olive oil) with lemon juice and a small amount of potassium hydroxide. They were able to create stone like structures which hardened if air dried at room temperature.

The researchers concluded that the so called stones seen after a gallbladder flush are the result of the mixing of olive oil with lemon juice (which is high in potassium) and digestive enzymes.

It is possible that some very small gallstones do get flushed out of the gallbladder during a flush, due to the large volume of olive oil you would drink, which would cause a healthy gallbladder to contract powerfully. Although a dysfunctional gallbladder does not have the ability to contract as well.

Chapter *Five*

Gallbladder remedies cheat sheet
- summary of the most important points

This chapter contains the most important remedies in this book, summarized for easy reference.

> *We would like you to read every page of this book, so you have a clear understanding of why you developed a gallbladder problem*

This will hopefully motivate you to make the required long term changes to your diet and lifestyle necessary if you want to get well. The rationale for our recommendations in this chapter is explained elsewhere in this book. This chapter merely summarizes the key points.

Symptoms of a gallbladder attack

- Intense pain in the right upper part of the abdomen
- Sometimes the pain radiates to the back of the right shoulder blade
- Nausea, with possible vomiting
- There may be burping or flatulence
- There may be fever and sweating
- A gallbladder attack most commonly occurs in the evening, around 2 hours after dinner.

Symptoms of a gallbladder attack usually last between one and four hours.

First aid remedies for alleviating the pain and reducing the duration of a gallbladder attack

- Sip on warm peppermint tea or flaxseed tea. See recipes on page 58.
- Sip on half a glass of warm water with half a teaspoon of Magnesium Ultra Potent powder.
- Sip on warm water containing a small amount of apple cider vinegar or fresh lemon juice.
- Lie down in bed and apply a hot pack or a castor oil hot pack. See instructions on page 56.

Strategies for reducing the risk of a gallbladder attack and staying out of hospital

- Don't overeat. Eat smaller meals more frequently.
- Don't eat too much fat in one go, but conversely don't follow a low fat diet because that would make your gallstones worse over the long term.
- Avoid the danger foods that can trigger a gallbladder attack; they include dairy products, gluten, eggs, onions, sugar and pork. There may be others; you will need to determine which foods cause problems for you.
- Take an ox bile supplement to raise the amount of bile in your digestive tract since your poor, struggling gallbladder cannot secrete sufficient levels.

Good foods	Bad foods
Eat more	*Eat less or avoid altogether*
Beet leaves	Dairy products - eg. milk, cheese, yogurt
Beets	
Chicory	Gluten - wheat, rye, oats, barley, spelt
Endive	Sugar
Dandelion leaves	Eggs
Globe artichoke	Onions
Radishes - red and daikon	Pork
Lemons and limes	Polyunsaturated vegetable oil derived from most seeds and nuts
Turmeric - fresh rhizome or dried and ground	
All vegetables - except potatoes	Margarine and non-dairy spread
All fruit but limit to two serves a day	Gluten free foods (bread, pasta, etc.) should be avoided or kept to a minimum
Fish and other seafood	
Poultry	
Red meat	
- preferably grass fed	
Good fats - avocados, olive, macadamia, avocado or coconut oil	
Fresh herbs (arugula, basil, watercress)	
Cabbage	
Kale	

Nuts, seeds and legumes can be eaten in small quantities if you feel you can digest them well. If you suffer with irritable bowel syndrome or several food allergies, it is best to avoid these foods for now while your digestive system is healing. Some people are able to digest nuts better if they have been soaked beforehand or ground in a food processor or coffee grinder.

Most important supplements for gallstones

- A liver tonic containing the herbs St Mary's thistle, dandelion, taurine and globe artichoke, taken twice daily with meals. I recommend the liver tonic called Livatone.

- An ox bile supplement. Take one ox bile capsule at the beginning of each meal.

- Apple cider vinegar - one tablespoon in ¼ cup warm water five minutes before meals, plus use it as a salad dressing with extra virgin olive oil, macadamia nut oil or avocado oil.

- Taurine and glycine - 1000 to 2000mg of each per day, taken with food.

- Magnesium and malic acid supplement. One teaspoon of powder in water or juice per day with a meal. *Avoid magnesium supplements that contain magnesium oxide because it is poorly absorbed and can cause digestive upsets.* Better absorbed forms of magnesium are magnesium amino acid chelate, magnesium diglycinate, magnesium ascorbate, magnesium orotate and magnesium phosphate.

  Avoid magnesium supplements that contain calcium, as this can compete for absorption with the magnesium.

- Vitamin C - 2 grams twice daily with or without food.

- Digestive enzymes and hydrochloric acid (betaine hydrochloride), as found in Super Digestive Enzymes supplement if you have symptoms of indigestion such as bloating, gas or burping. Take them in the middle of meals.

- Glutamine powder if you suffer with irritable bowel syndrome, bloating or diarrhea. Dose is 2 grams twice daily away from food.

If you have any questions about our recommendations please phone our nutritional advisors on 1888 755 4837.

Chapter Six

Basic structure and function of the gallbladder

In this section we will briefly explain where your gallbladder is and how it functions. This will give you a greater understanding of why gallbladder problems occur in the first place, thus helping you to restore your gallbladder health.

The gallbladder

The gallbladder is a small, sac-like organ that is approximately 3 inches (eight centimeters) long and 1.5 inches (four centimeters) wide. It sits behind the liver, in the upper right segment of your abdomen, roughly at the level of your lowest right rib.

The walls of the gallbladder are composed of smooth muscle, which allows the gallbladder to contract forcefully in order to squirt bile into the common bile duct and then into your small intestine during a meal. Your gallbladder really behaves like a squirt gun.

Your gallbladder has two main functions: to store bile and to concentrate bile, so that it becomes more potent by the time it is needed. Generally bile is concentrated five-fold while stored in the gallbladder. As you can see, the gallbladder is merely a sac for storing and ejecting bile, so it cannot take the blame for gallstone formation or inflammation.

It is the health of your liver that is the biggest determinant in whether or not you will develop gallbladder disease, as the liver determines the quality of bile produced and whether or not that bile leads to stone formation

Bile

Bile is a brownish green liquid that has three important functions in the body:

1. Bile contains bile acids which act as an emulsifier or detergent, critical for the digestion and absorption of fats and fat soluble vitamins in the small intestine. Bile basically breaks fat molecules into smaller globules, so that digestive enzymes (lipases) can act to break them down, making them ready for absorption. Bile acids are also known as bile salts.

2. Bile is an excretion route for many wastes and toxins that need elimination from the body. These wastes enter the small intestine in the bile and are then eliminated in feces. Bilirubin is the breakdown product of red blood cells and it forms a major component of bile. Your body excretes excess fat and fat soluble toxins as well as hormone residues through bile.

3. Bile deodorises the stool, gives it its brown color and has a gentle laxative effect. People with overly smelly feces often do not secrete enough bile. Constipated people often do not produce enough bile either. In fact in most instances a sluggish bowel is due to a sluggish liver that is not producing sufficient good quality bile.

The average person's liver produces between 13½ and 27 ounces (400 and 800 mL) of bile each day. Liver cells (hepatocytes) produce bile and secrete it into tiny tubes within the liver called canaliculi. From there, the bile travels into bile ducts within the liver. At this stage bile contains large quantities of bile acids and cholesterol.

As bile travels through the bile ducts of the liver, it is modified by the addition of a bicarbonate rich watery solution, secreted by the liver cells that line the bile ducts. Bile then travels into the gallbladder where it is stored and concentrated, ready to be secreted into the intestines during a meal.

When the bile is being concentrated in the gallbladder, 90 percent of the water in it gets rebsorbed. That leaves only approximately a few tablespoons of concentrated bile, ready to be ejected when needed. The amount of bile your gallbladder ejects during meal depends on several factors, including how thick the bile is (thick bile doesn't squirt out as easily) and how well the walls of your gallbladder are able to contract.

The role of bile in healthy digestion

Knowing how the gallbladder functions will help you understand which foods are beneficial for gallbladder health and which foods you are better off avoiding. If you've had a long standing gallbladder problem you'll learn how to minimize the risk of a full blown gallbladder attack.

Bile is an alkaline fluid with a pH between 7.6 and 8.6. Bile acids are a major component of bile and they are actually made from cholesterol.

Cholesterol is a very valuable substance that has numerous beneficial effects in your body; this is merely one of them. You need cholesterol in order to have efficient fat digestion. Most of the cholesterol in your body was made in your liver. In the production of bile, cholesterol is converted into the bile acids cholic and chenodeoxycholic acids, which are then bound to the amino acids glycine or taurine.

After this occurs, the bile acids are said to be conjugated and ready to be used. Glycine and taurine are therefore very important for the production of healthy bile in individuals with gallstones or excessively thick and sludgy bile.

Bile production is actually the major way your body gets rid of excess cholesterol it no longer requires. Your liver converts an average of 500 milligrams of cholesterol into bile acids each day. The bile eventually enters your intestines and some of it is eliminated from your body in bowel actions. However if you are constipated you will not be excreting cholesterol efficiently. Too much of the cholesterol will get reabsorbed back into your bloodstream and then end up back at your liver.

This is why having regular and efficient bowel habits is an important strategy in maintaining a healthy cholesterol level

Bile secretion in fat digestion

Bile is required for fat digestion, therefore if you have not eaten for some time, bile tends to stay in your gallbladder where it is concentrated. A small amount of bile will trickle out of your gallbladder, along the common bile duct on its way to your small intestine. Before emptying into your small intestine, the bile duct passes through your pancreas. This is important to remember because it is possible for a gallstone to become trapped in the duct within the pancreas, causing an acute case of pancreatitis. This is a medical emergency and is covered in greater detail on page 94.

To prevent bile from continually trickling into your small intestine, a valve at the end of the common bile duct remains closed between meals, preventing bile from entering the small intestine. This valve is called the Sphincter of Oddi or the hepatopancreatic sphincter and it prevents both bile and pancreatic digestive enzymes from entering the small intestine between meals when they are not required.

This diagram (right) shows the location of the gallbladder and how bile travels through the bile ducts.

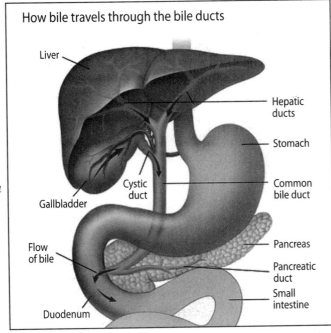

How bile travels through the bile ducts

Liver

Hepatic ducts

Stomach

Cystic duct

Common bile duct

Gallbladder

Flow of bile

Pancreas

Pancreatic duct

Small intestine

Duodenum

When food that contains some fat enters the first part of your small intestine (duodenum), just below your stomach, cells lining your small intestine secrete a hormone called CCK into your bloodstream. The full name of this hormone is cholecystokinin but it's commonly abbreviated to CCK. The word is derived from Greek - chole refers to bile, cysto refers to sac and kinin means move. So the word means move the bile sac.

This hormone triggers your gallbladder to contract and it makes the sphincter of Oddi open up, allowing bile to enter the small intestine. CCK also triggers the pancreas to release its digestive enzymes into your small intestine.

When bile enters your small intestine, it acts like a detergent, helping to break the fat globules into smaller molecules, so that they can be completely digested by enzymes. Fat digesting enzymes are called lipases. Most of the fats that get digested in your small intestine do not get absorbed into your bloodstream like other nutrients, vitamins and minerals you have consumed. Most fats get absorbed directly into your lymphatic system, and from there get carried in lymphatic vessels to your heart. This makes sense because fat is a rich energy source and is actually the preferred energy source for your hard working heart muscle.

Long chain fatty acids that you consume in your diet must first be emulsified by bile, then digested by lipases and then absorbed into your lymphatic system. However, short chain fatty acids, and some medium chain fatty acids do not require bile for their digestion. They get absorbed directly into the bloodstream and are taken straight to the liver. Coconut oil is mostly made up of the medium chain fatty acid lauric acid. It does not require bile for digestion, and therefore does not place a strain on the gallbladder in individuals with compromised gallbladder function.

Chapter Seven

What goes wrong - why do gallstones form?

If an excessively high level of cholesterol and other fats is present in the bile, the bile will become too concentrated, thick and sludgy.

Gallstones form when the cholesterol in bile reaches a point of super saturation. This means no more cholesterol can dissolve in the bile. If any more cholesterol is added to the bile, it will precipitate and form a solid residue. The solid cholesterol residue starts out as tiny molecules the size of grains of sand, but this is the beginning of gallstone formation.

Gallstones form when too much cholesterol enters the bile and/or not enough bile acids are present in the bile to keep the bile fluid and thin. When too much cholesterol and other fats are present in the bile, the bile becomes thicker and harder to squirt out whenever the gallbladder contracts. Over time, this excessively thick bile that has remained in your gallbladder too long, may start to form stones.

Thick and stagnant bile - a recipe for stone formation

When there is too much fat in your bile, the bile becomes a lot thicker and doesn't flow as freely.

A thick liquid always moves a lot more slowly than a thin watery fluid. Thick bile doesn't squirt out of your gallbladder the way it is supposed to when your gallbladder contracts. Therefore, if the bile in your gallbladder is excessively thick, each time your gallbladder contracts, less bile will flow out and more will be left behind.

This means less bile will enter your intestines every time you eat a meal that contains fat. That means you'll probably have symptoms of poor fat digestion, such as bloating, burping, nausea, possibly diarrhea after a fatty meal and possibly discomfort over the right side of your upper abdomen after a big meal. It also means gallstones are probably forming and growing inside your gallbladder.

If some bile is always left behind and not ejected from your gallbladder when it contracts, that bile becomes more and more concentrated.

Over time, more and more of the bile becomes sludge-like and prone to forming stones. As the bile in your gallbladder becomes thicker and thicker, less of it will leave your gallbladder as it contracts in response to a meal. This worsens the problem of cholesterol super-saturation and means stones will almost certainly form inside the gallbladder.

So you can see that the gallbladder itself is not to blame for stone formation; rather it is the excessively thick bile inside the gallbladder that is at fault

Sludge is the forerunner to gallstones.

Having excessively thick bile inside the gallbladder makes it much more difficult for the gallbladder to contract properly and expel all the bile that's inside. Therefore stagnant bile is never able to leave your gallbladder. It remains there indefinitely and predictably eventually forms gallstones.

If you don't address the dietary, digestive and metabolic factors that cause gallstones to form in the first place, this scenario will only get worse.

Gallstones can become so large or numerous that they interfere with the ability of the gallbladder to function properly.

This can occur for two reasons:

1. Gallstones are hard and can cause mechanical irritation to the lining of the gallbladder.

2. Because gallstones take up space, they can actually prevent the gallbladder from being able to contract properly and expel bile from within it.

The factors mentioned above can cause pain and irritation but they can also cause permanent changes to the gallbladder itself; most commonly thickening of the walls of the gallbladder and gallbladder polyps.

Chapter Eight

Diagnosis of gallbladder disease

Ultrasound

An ultrasound is the standard way to diagnose gallstones. In most instances, a patient sees their doctor regarding recurring pain or discomfort in the right upper portion of the abdomen, which prompts the doctor to order an ultrasound.

An ultrasound is a fast and risk free method of detecting gallstones. It can show the quantity and size of gallstones, and their location within the gallbladder. Getting periodic ultrasounds of your gallbladder is a good way to keep track of the progress you make in shrinking or dissolving any gallstones.

An ultrasound can show you if your gallbladder is inflamed, if the walls have thickened and if there are other abnormalities such as polyps or a tumor in the gallbladder

An ultrasound can also give you an idea of the diameter of your common bile duct. It's good to know how wide your common bile duct is in relation to the stones in your gallbladder. You will know if you're at risk of getting a stone trapped in the duct while on its way to your intestine. An X ray is not used to diagnose gallstones because only around ten percent of gallstones can be seen on an X ray. However, this test will sometimes still be performed if your doctor suspects there are other complicating factors involved.

ERCP (Endoscopic Retrograde Cholangiopancreatography)

This test is used if it is suspected there is a stone in your bile duct or to remove a stone that may be trapped there. A flexible tube called an endoscope is passed into your mouth, down past the stomach and into the first past of the small intestine. A dye is injected into the common bile duct and then an X ray is taken to see if there are any blockages in the bile duct. If a stone is present, it can be removed during this procedure. There are some risks associated with this procedure, the worst one being pancreatitis. Some people may be allergic to the dye that is used in this procedure.

HIDA scan

A HIDA scan is a way of checking how well your gallbladder functions. HIDA stands for Hepatobiliary Iminodiacetic acid scan and it creates pictures of your liver, gallbladder, bile ducts and small intestine. This test uses a small and harmless amount of radiation. A radioactive chemical, or tracer is used, which highlights the flow of bile from the liver, via the bile ducts, gallbladder and then to the small intestine.

Your doctor may order a HIDA scan to check for the following abnormalities:

- Gallstones
- A poorly functioning gallbladder
- Inflammation in the gallbladder (cholecystitis)
- Blockage of the bile ducts
- Leakage of bile
- Congenital abnormalities in the bile ducts

A HIDA scan can detect biliary dyskinesia, which is a motility disorder of the biliary system. It basically means a low functioning gallbladder. Biliary dyskinesia is usually a forerunner to gallstone formation.

This test can also measure the rate at which bile is ejected from your gallbladder, thus checking how well it is able to contract. This is known as the gallbladder ejection fraction.

A normal ejection fraction is between 35 and 75 percent. That means, when your gallbladder contracts during a meal, it is supposed to squirt out between 35 and 75 percent of its bile into your small intestine. If it squirts significantly less, it means not enough bile will enter your intestines at each meal for good digestion, and more bile will remain in your gallbladder, encouraging the formation and growth of stones.

A normal ejection fraction is considered to be more than 40 percent.

If your reading is less than 35 percent and you are in considerable discomfort regularly, your doctor will probably advise you to have your gallbladder removed.

How this test is performed

You will be asked to fast for at least two hours before the test.

A radioactive tracer will be injected into a vein in your arm. The tracer travels to your liver and is absorbed by the bile-producing cells of your liver. The tracer travels with the bile made in your liver, into your gallbladder, then through your bile ducts and into your small intestine.

While this is happening, a scanner will take pictures of your abdomen, highlighting the flow of bile as it moves through your body. The hormone CCK (cholecystokinin) is also injected into your vein in order to stimulate gallbladder contractions.

The test takes approximately an hour.

The radioactive tracer injected into your arm takes one to two days to leave your body completely. Therefore you are encouraged to drink plenty of water to flush it from your body sooner, flush the toilet twice after using it and wash your hands thoroughly afterwards. It is also best to limit close contact with children.

A HIDA scan is not recommended for pregnant or breastfeeding women.

Along with giving you a reading for your gallbladder ejection fraction, the HIDA scan will also tell you how quickly the radioactive tracer moved through your hepatobiliary system.

If the tracer moved too slowly, it can indicate a blockage or obstruction in a bile duct, or a problem in the liver. If the radioactive tracer cannot be seen in your gallbladder, this usually indicates inflammation of the gallbladder (cholecystitis). If the tracer is detected in areas where it shouldn't be, this usually indicates leakage of the biliary ducts.

What should you do if you have a low gallbladder ejection fraction?

It is commonly recommended that people with a low gallbladder ejection fraction, and symptoms of gallbladder disease should have their gallbladder removed. Your doctor probably thinks "Well, your gallbladder doesn't seem to be contracting properly, you're in pain, so you may as well get it taken out". This is not always the best advice.

Let's look at two possible scenarios:

1. If there are stones in your gallbladder and you have been in considerable discomfort for some time, and you have suffered more than one serious gallbladder attack, it may be necessary to have your gallbladder removed. We have discussed when it is advisable to have your gallbladder removed in detail on page 93.

2. If there are no stones in your gallbladder, but you experience pain or discomfort and you have a low ejection fraction, it is definitely best to try and keep your gallbladder.

   You need to fix your digestion and that should improve the ability of your gallbladder to contract. It will also reduce the inflammation in your gallbladder that causes the pain or discomfort. Food allergy or intolerance is a very common cause of functional gallbladder problems and we have discussed this topic in chapter two.

Blood tests

A blood test cannot diagnose a gallbladder condition, but it can give us an idea of the severity of the gallbladder problem and whether an infection or other complicating factors are present.

The following blood tests should be performed:

Full blood count

The purpose of this test is to check the quantity of white blood cells in your bloodstream.

Elevated white blood cells usually indicate an infection. In this case white cells called neutrophils may be elevated and this is referred to as neutrophilia. Sometimes the white blood cells called leukocytes can be elevated if there is inflammation of the gallbladder (cholecystitis), and this is called leucocytosis.

ESR (erythrocyte sedimentation rate) and CRP (C-reactive protein)

These tests are indicators of inflammation in your body. These markers are usually elevated during infections or acute inflammation.

Liver function test

This test checks the levels of enzymes in your liver and can indicate whether there is inflammation or cell damage in your liver. It can also indicate whether the flow of bile through your liver has been blocked (bile stasis).

The liver enzyme ALP (alkaline phosphatase) is most commonly elevated in bile stasis. This is because this enzyme is found in the cells lining the biliary ducts within the liver. However, ALP is also present in bones and the placenta and levels typically rise two to three times normal in the third trimester of pregnancy.

A liver function test also checks your blood bilirubin level. During a gallbladder attack some people become jaundiced, which means the whites of their eyes may turn yellow.

If the flow of bile has become obstructed by a stone or due to inflammation, bile can leak into the bloodstream. Therefore during an acute gallbladder attack you may have a high blood level of conjugated bilirubin.

Pancreatic enzymes

You may have a blood test to check your level of pancreatic enzymes, in order to check for inflammation of your pancreas (pancreatitis). Amylase and lipase are the names of the enzymes found in the pancreas that may leak into the bloodstream if the pancreas becomes inflamed.

The most common cause of pancreatitis is an inflamed gallbladder, and pancreatitis can be a life threatening disease, so it is wise to check your pancreas if you've had a gallbladder attack.

What if it's not your gallbladder after all?

Other conditions that present with similar symptoms to gallbladder disease

If you suffer with the symptoms of gallbladder disease listed on page 17 please see your doctor for an accurate diagnosis. There is a possibility you might be suffering with one or more of the following conditions:

- Peptic ulcer (ulcer in the stomach or small intestine)
- Irritable bowel syndrome (IBS). This is usually caused by food intolerance and our recommendations in chapter two should greatly help you.
- Hepatitis
- Pancreatitis
- Fatty liver with liver congestion
- Cancer of an abdominal organ - such as pancreatic cancer, intestinal cancer, liver cancer, stomach cancer or cancer of the gallbladder or biliary ducts.
- Autoimmune disease - such as autoimmune hepatitis, sclerosing cholangitis or primary biliary cirrhosis

- Stomach inflammation known as gastritis – this may be caused by infection with bacteria known as helicobacter pylori; these bacteria live in the stomach lining and flare up if you eat excess sugar or excess carbohydrate
- Reflux of acid from the stomach back into the esophagus
- Food allergies
- Gluten intolerance
- Liver cysts caused by sluggish bile flow (these are often small)
- Severe emotional stress causing spasm in the smooth muscle in the gut
- Adverse drug reactions from anti-inflammatory drugs which can upset the liver and stomach

Chapter *Nine*

The conventional medical treatment of gallstones

The most common medical solution for gallstones is to remove the gallbladder. In fact, this is one of the most commonly performed hospital procedures today, and a gallbladder attack is one of the most common reasons for hospital admission due to abdominal pain. There are some other alternatives to gallbladder surgery, and we will describe them in the following section.

Cholecystectomy (removal of the gallbladder)

In the past, removal of the gallbladder was a major surgery, where a large section of the abdomen was opened up. That meant there was a significant risk of complication and patients were at high risk of post-surgical infections.

> *Approximately 25 years ago laparoscopic surgery (keyhole surgery) was introduced, and since then gallbladder surgery became a much faster and simpler operation*

Patients with a high degree of inflammation in their gallbladder (cholecystitis) along with multiple gallstones and regular, severe symptoms should have their gallbladder taken out sooner, rather than later. This is because there is a higher risk of complications such as infections and pancreatitis in people with a highly inflamed gallbladder.

In those instances keyhole surgery usually cannot be performed, and the operation becomes a riskier procedure with a longer recovery time.

During laparoscopic gallbladder surgery, a very small incision is made in your abdomen and a small, flexible telescope with a surgical instrument at the end of it is inserted inside. The surgeon will look at your gallbladder on a computer screen and remove it with the tiny surgical instrument through a very small incision.

Recovery time is fairly fast for most people and there is a minimal risk of infection.

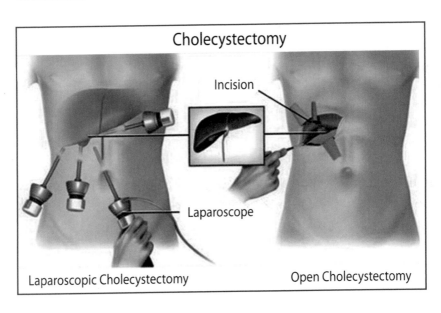

Cholecystectomy

Incision

Laparoscope

Laparoscopic Cholecystectomy

Open Cholecystectomy

A cholangiogram is performed at the time of surgery in order to make sure no stones are blocked in a bile duct and that the bile duct hasn't been damaged. A cholangiogram is an X ray that uses a contrast medium (dye) in order to visualize the bile ducts adequately.

Potential problems with cholecystectomy

These are the main problems with having the gallbladder removed:

- Your gallbladder is gone but your pain is still there. According to a study published in the British Journal of General Practice, one third of the patients who had their gallbladder removed saw their doctor again with the same pain they had suffered prior to the surgery. [20.]

Sometimes the pain or discomfort isn't caused by the stones; it may be caused by inflammation in the bile ducts within the liver, or the common bile duct between the liver and the small intestine. Sometimes the pain is caused by a fatty liver or indigestion, or inflammation in the stomach or another abdominal organ. This is why it is essential to have a thorough investigation if you experience the types of symptoms we have described on page 17.

Your doctor may discover that you have gallstones, but it's possible that you have another health problem, and that ailment is responsible for your pain, not the gallstones.

- Your gallbladder has been removed and you are no longer in pain; however now you regularly experience digestive problems such as diarrhea after an oily meal and a general inability to digest fats.

Symptoms of indigestion common after gallbladder removal are urgent and loose stools, abdominal bloating, nausea and burping. Some people do not experience any of these symptoms and they are the lucky ones. However, everybody who has had their gallbladder removed will not be able to digest fats adequately and this almost guarantees they will develop deficiencies of essential fatty acids and fat soluble vitamins.

This topic is covered in great detail in chapter eleven.

- If you have lost your gallbladder, you are at greater risk of developing a fatty liver, stones in the bile ducts within your liver (which are much more difficult to treat) and liver cysts.

ERCP (Endoscopic retrograde cholangiopancreatography)

This procedure is usually used for removing a stone caught in a bile duct. Sometimes an ultrasound cannot detect a stone in a bile duct. If your doctor suspects this may be a problem for you, an ERCP can detect a stone as well as remove it. An endoscope is passed through the mouth, down through the stomach and to the point in the small intestine where the common bile duct empties.

A dye is squirted into the common bile duct to visualize if there are any blockages. If a stone is present, a surgical tool can be passed along the endoscope in order to remove it.

Non-surgical medical treatments for gallstones

Lithotripsy

The full name of this procedure is Extracorporeal shockwave lithotripsy (ESWL). This is where ultrasound waves are used to break up stones in the gallbladder. This procedure is only suitable for small, solitary stones.

Lithotripsy is rarely performed because the stones tend to come back fairly quickly. This is to be expected if none of the factors that promoted the stones to grow in the first place are addressed. In fact, according to research approximately 45 percent of patients who underwent lithotripsy eventually had their gallbladder taken out because the problem recurred. [21.]

Antibiotics are usually given prophylactically to patients who have had lithotripsy because there is the risk of a small stone fragment getting stuck in the bile duct and causing an infection.

Oral bile salt therapy

This involves taking medication to dissolve gallstones. This method is only used for small non-calcified gallstones. Small stones usually means less than 1.5 centimeters in diameter.

Calcified gallstones have been in the gallbladder a lot longer, they are harder and take much longer to dissolve. This method is rarely used by most doctors because it is a very slow process and stones tend to return. Therefore it usually only gets recommended to people who can't have surgery for one reason or another.

If you combine this method with our recommendations in chapter two, you should get quite good results

This method works by increasing the amount of bile acids in your bile and reducing the amount of cholesterol in your bile. Over time, this helps to thin the bile and slowly dissolve the stones that are present.

The most commonly used drug to dissolve gallstones is ursodeoxycholic acid, which is sold under the brand names Ursofalk, Ursodiol or Actigal. This is a very safe medication, because really it's a natural bile salt that your own liver produces, but may not be producing enough of at the moment.

It can help to reduce the risk of gallbladder pain and an acute gallbladder attack. Not many doctors use it these days because it works slowly and gallstones redevelop in most people. However, if you are motivated to change your diet and follow our guidelines in chapter two, ursodeoxychlic acid can be a valuable part of your treatment plan. This medication can help to reduce indigestion and itchy skin associated with elevated blood bilirubin. It is synthesised in a laboratory; it does not come from the bile of an animal.

Ursodiol can also be used to prevent the formation of gallstones, especially in patients who are undergoing rapid weight loss.

Normally in the gallbladder, there is a balance between bile salts and cholesterol and fast weight loss can cause this balance to be disturbed. During fast weight loss (more than 1.4 kilograms or 3 pounds per week), bile salts tend to decrease and cholesterol increases.

Ursodiol is also used as a treatment for primary biliary cirrhosis (PBC), which is a liver disease that destroys the liver's bile ducts. When this happens, bile cannot flow to the small intestine to help with the digestion of fat. The bile remains trapped in the liver and causes damage to the liver's cells which can lead to cirrhosis. Since Ursodiol is a bile acid, it improves liver function in those with PBC. It can increase life expectancy and buy time for the patient who is waiting for a liver transplant.

Ursodiol must be taken daily for life or until the transplant occurs.

Cholestyramine

This is another type of oral medication that can be used to help dissolve gallstones. It is sold under the brand name Questran Lite. It is usually used to lower cholesterol levels and works by binding bile salts in the bowel and taking them out of the body in the stool. It is a safe, effective and well tolerated medication.

Cholestyramine can relieve the awful itching that some people with gallbladder disease experience because of elevated blood bilirubin level. This occurs if there is bile obstruction within the liver or biliary system. Cholestryamine is very effective in controlling chronic diarrhea that can be a side effect of gallbladder removal. It is taken in sachets as it is a powder. Unfortunately Questran sachets contain the artificial sweetener aspartame, but that's hardly surprising from a drug company.

Because it reduces cholesterol, cholestyramine also reduces the absorption of fat soluble vitamins, including vitamins K, D, E and A, fat soluble antioxidants such as carotenoids and lycopene, as well as essential fatty acids. This is the biggest disadvantage of this medication.

Chapter Ten

Sometimes it has to go!

Signs and symptoms that indicate your gallbladder should come out

In this book we have emphasised how important the gallbladder is to overall health and how far too many people lose their gallbladder when a few simple diet changes could have prevented that. Unfortunately, sometimes it really is too late and it's actually safer to have the gallbladder removed.

> *Leaving a very diseased gallbladder inside you is asking for trouble because it's possible to develop some very serious and life threatening complications*

Please do not solely rely on the information in this book for the management of your gallbladder condition. It is very important that you are regularly monitored by your doctor, in order to avoid harmful consequences.

A severe gallbladder attack can cause the gallbladder or a bile duct to rupture. It can also produce acute pancreatitis, which can be life threatening.

Most gallbladder attacks last between one and four hours. If you have had several in the past, you will be familiar with how long they last for you, the nature of the pain and what works to relieve the pain.

If you have a gallbladder attack that lasts longer than usual, the pain is more severe and the pain does not respond to your usual self help strategies, please go to a hospital immediately.

If in doubt, please seek medical care as soon as possible.

Sometimes the walls of the gallbladder become extremely thickened (hypertrophied) to the point where the gallbladder can no longer contract properly at all. Sometimes the walls of the gallbladder become calcified, and this also inhibits normal contraction. These conditions, as well as infection of the gallbladder are clear signs that you are better off having your gallbladder removed.

Potential complications of gallstones

The following conditions are all potential complications of gallstones:

- acute gallbladder attack
- obstructive jaundice This is where the flow of bile becomes blocked and therefore bilirubin leaks into the bloodstream. Jaundice can cause yellowing of the eyes and skin, itchy skin, pale, tan-colored stools and dark colored urine.
- infection of the gallbladder
- acute pancreatitis. The gallbladder lies very close to the pancreas and inflammation or infection of the gallbladder can easily inflame the pancreas. Sometimes a stone from the gallbladder moves out and gets trapped in the pancreatic duct. Acute pancreatitis is a medical emergency and causes extreme pain, nausea, vomiting and fever. Acute pancreatitis results in a swift trip to hospital.
- acute cholangitis. This is inflammation of the bile duct (tube that carries the bile from the gallbladder to the small intestine). The inflammation can be caused by a trapped stone or by infection due to a lodged stone.
- gallstone ileus. This is bowel obstruction caused by a gallstone.

If you have had several gallbladder attacks, you are in pain or discomfort after nearly every meal, you have stones in your gallbladder and a poor HIDA scan result (meaning your gallbladder cannot contract properly), you should probably have your gallbladder removed.

It is best not to hang out too long avoiding surgery because if you are admitted to hospital suffering one of the above complications, you will not be a candidate for keyhole (laparoscopic) surgery. Instead, you'll have an open cholecystectomy, which carries more risks and will leave you with a much longer hospital stay and longer recovery period. You will also not be able to choose your doctor or hospital if you are admitted to emergency.

Other conditions affecting the gallbladder or bile ducts

Most of this book has focused on gallstones and inflammation of the gallbladder because they are certainly the most common gallbladder conditions. There are other things that can go wrong with the gallbladder; sometimes they occur in isolation and sometimes they are present along with stones.

The vast majority of the recommendations in this book are equally applicable to the conditions described below.

Gallbladder polyps

Polyps in the gallbladder usually do not cause any symptoms and are generally discovered incidentally during an upper abdominal ultrasound. If one or more polyps have been found in your gallbladder, you should have another ultrasound in three to six months to check if they've increased in size. Gallbladder polyps should not have increased in size significantly after that time, however a cancerous growth would have increased significantly.

Some doctors recommend the gallbladder be removed if a polyp is greater than one centimeter in size because of the risk it may turn cancerous. It's probably best to just keep monitoring it with ultrasounds and follow the recommendations in chapter two but this depends on your individual case, so please be monitored by your own doctor. If you have gallbladder polyps, we recommend you avoid gluten and dairy products and take a selenium and vitamin D supplement. The optimal dose of selenium is between 200 and 300 micrograms daily.

Gallbladder cancer

This is not a common cancer in the United States. Just like with all gallbladder problems, women are more susceptible than men.

Cancer begins in the cells lining the inside of the gallbladder, and as it grows it spreads outwards. Gallbladder cancer is often not detected until it's quite advanced because the symptoms can be vague and mild or entirely non-existent. This means the prognosis is often poor.

There are several known risk factors for gallbladder cancer including:

- Chronic infection of the gallbladder
- A history of gallstones, especially mixed stones. That means some of the stones in the gallbladder are made of cholesterol and some are pigment stones.
- Obesity
- High sugar and carbohydrate diet
- Women who have had several children are at greater risk than women who have never had any children.

Sometimes cancer can form in the bile ducts themselves. Chronic infection is also a risk factor for this type of cancer.

The underlying message is don't leave a chronic gallbladder infection untreated

This type of cancer is most likely to occur in individuals who have suffered with a sick gallbladder for many years that should have been surgically removed. [22.] You can reduce your risk of gallbladder cancer by not allowing a gallbladder infection to go untreated, and by taking supplemental selenium and vitamin D.

Why do the walls of the gallbladder become thickened?

The walls of the gallbladder can get thickened if one or more stones have been there for a long time. The stones are irritating to the wall of the gallbladder, and the gallbladder must contract more forcefully if there are stones inside. Celiac disease and food intolerance can disrupt the ability of the gallbladder to contract properly, and this can eventually lead to thickened walls.

Porcelain gallbladder

This describes a condition where the walls of the gallbladder have become calcified and hard. Chronic inflammation of the walls of the gallbladder leads to eventual scarring and this can promote the deposition of calcium. It is usually a sign of long standing gallbladder problems. Because of the calcification, sometimes the gallbladder cannot be seen on ultrasound.

Sclerosing cholangitis

This is an autoimmune disease that causes the bile ducts to harden, obstructing the normal flow of bile. Both the bile ducts within the liver and those outside the liver become inflamed, which eventually leads to scarring and hardening of the ducts. Obstruction to the normal flow of bile causes the build up and stasis of bile within the liver, which can damage the liver. Symptoms of sclerosing cholangitis include jaundice, itching of the skin and tenderness in the right upper abdomen. Our recommendations for sclerosing cholangitis and primary biliary cirrhosis are the same, which we outline below.

Primary biliary cirrhosis

This is an autoimmune liver disease that causes progressive destruction of the bile ducts within the liver. This causes bile to build up in the liver (cholestasis), which damages the liver.

Sclerosing cholangitis and primary biliary cirrhosis are serious diseases that must receive prompt treatment and regular monitoring in order to avoid significant destruction of the liver. Ursofalk (ursodeoxycholic acid) is the prescription medicine that helps to dissolve gallstones and it is given to patients with these diseases because it helps to reduce inflammation within the liver. Steroids and immunosuppressants are also usually prescribed for these conditions because they are autoimmune.

The nutritional treatment of these conditions is quite complex because of the serious nature of these conditions.

A gluten and dairy free diet is mandatory and additional food sensitivities are often also present

The focus of treatment is to improve digestive, immune and liver health. The most important nutritional supplements are vitamin D, selenium, glutamine and a probiotic (good bowel bacteria). A liver tonic containing the herbs St Mary's thistle, dandelion, globe artichoke and taurine is most beneficial. This supplement is called Livatone. For more information please call us in the USA on 1888 755 4837 or see www.liverdoctor.com

People with inflammation in and/or around their bile ducts would also benefit from taking a supplement called N-acetyl cysteine (NAC). This is a form of the sulfur containing amino acid cysteine, which is a precursor of glutathione. Glutathione is a powerful antioxidant that enables your liver to detoxify your bloodstream. Glutathione helps to mop up free radicals in your body and it has strong anti-inflammatory actions. That makes NAC extremely beneficial for all autoimmune diseases of the liver and bile ducts. N-acetyl cysteine supplements raise the level of glutathione in liver cells.

The stress of chronic liver disease depletes glutathione and this is why supplementing with one of its precursors, NAC helps to protect against ongoing liver damage. Selenium is also required for glutathione production and that's why it is also so critical for autoimmune disease. A good dose of selenium is between 200 and 300 micrograms daily.

Liver fluke

Liver fluke disease is a chronic parasitic disease of the bile ducts. Infection with this parasite occurs through eating fluke-infested, fresh-water raw fish. The most common types of liver flukes are *Clonorchis sinensis, Opisthorchis viverrini and Opisthorchis felineus.*

Approximately 35 million people are infected with liver flukes throughout the world and the very high incidence of cancer of the bile ducts (cholangiocarcinoma) in some countries is associated with a high prevalence of liver fluke infection.

It is most common in South-East Asia, South Korea, Taiwan, Northern Vietnam, Laos and Northeast Thailand, Eastern Europe Eastern Russia, Manchuria, Northern Siberia and China and 15 million Chinese people carry liver fluke. People living along rivers are prone to infection by flukes because they have a habit of eating raw or undercooked fresh-water fish.

Liver fluke is not common in the Western world and I have had two patients with this disease in Australia over 35 years of practising clinical medicine. In North American countries where many Asian immigrants are living, people may be infected and the diagnosis is often missed until severe liver damage has resulted.

This food-borne malady is an important public health issue and liver fluke infection does not receive the awareness it deserves.

The flukes get into the small bile ducts inside the liver and the gallbladder where they live for 20-30 years. The flukes cause chronic inflammation of the bile ducts causing scarring (fibrosis) of the bile ducts and bile duct dilatation.

Most people infected with this parasite have no symptoms however patients with severe infection suffer from fatigue and abdominal discomfort. Long standing infection may cause stone formation in the bile ducts and gallbladder, recurrent bacterial secondary infections in the bile ducts and cancer of the bile ducts.

Severe infection can cause an enlarged liver (hepatomegaly) and abdominal complaints such as abdominal pain, anorexia, nausea, vomiting and indigestion.

Jaundice is due to the mechanical obstruction in the bile ducts caused by a multitude of flukes in patients with a heavy infection, or it is due to bile duct obstruction caused by stones, or bile duct cancer (cholangiocarcinoma) as a late complication of chronic infection.

A liver fluke is a type of flat worm. One adult fluke lays 2000 - 4000 eggs each day and the eggs are excreted through the bile ducts and feces of the infected person. The cycle recirculates via eating of raw fresh-water fish.

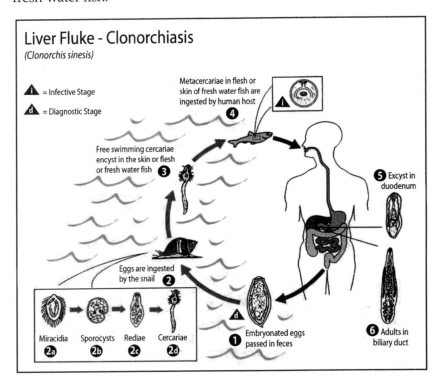

Testing Patients for Liver Fluke Infection

In endemic areas, it is recommended to do screening tests such as a stool ova test and a liver ultrasound scan. The high risk groups for liver fluke infection are those who have a history of eating raw, freshwater fish in endemic areas. If an ultrasound scan or CT images show dilatation of the bile ducts then anthelminthic drugs should be prescribed.

People should be told to have regular periodic stool tests to check for the presence of eggs in the stool. Also anyone who has travelled to these parts of the world and eaten raw or under cooked fish should be tested.

The typical appearance of past/healed liver fluke infection is widespread dilatation of the bile ducts inside the liver without evidence of an obstructing cause (dilatation without obstruction) on ultrasound, CT or MRI scans of the liver. This picture is frequently found in healthy looking but infected people in endemic areas.

The control of liver fluke and any food borne infections requires collaboration between the sectors of public health, the food industry and the media. Consumer education is crucial to make people aware of the need to stop eating raw fish. Because of more immigration and travel more doctors should know about the high prevalence of liver fluke infection among healthy looking people and the long term severe complications of the infection, especially the high risk of cancer and the need to closely monitor the patients longterm.

Important Point

If liver fluke is left undetected for years, this can become a very serious disease and cause destruction of the liver. Most people with liver fluke infection are completely unaware because they experience no symptoms at all. A small percentage of patients experience fatigue and non-specific abdominal discomfort, which easily gets mistaken for indigestion or irritable bowel syndrome. So it is important to have a high awareness of this insidious and destructive liver disease.

Medical treatment

Tablets are prescribed to kill the worms and these drugs are known as antihelmintic medications. If the disease is detected too late, sometimes the damage caused by the flukes is so extensive that a badly damaged part of the liver must be surgically removed. The sooner the infection is detected and eradicated, the less harm it is able to do to the bile ducts and the liver.

An experimental drug called tribendimidine could help cure millions of people infected with liver fluke. In a study published in The Lancet medical journal, researchers found that tribendimidine, is as safe and effective as the standard treatment for liver fluke. The standard treatment is a generic drug called praziquantel, which has a cure rate of 70 percent.

The cure rates for tribendimidine were much better than praziquantel, although this needs to be confirmed in larger clinical trials.

In contrast to the new drug, older drugs such as artemether, artesunate and mefloquine are not effective and should not be recommended for treating liver fluke.

Highest cure rates of 70 percent can be achieved in patients treated with tribendimidine, followed by 56 percent for those treated with praziquantel. Cure rates are much less from taking combined mefloquine and artesunate.

There are many types of parasitic worms and they cause disease in more than a billion people around the world. Over time these parasites have become increasingly resistant to available drugs; this brings an urgent need to find new drugs to fight them.

Flukes are very hard to eradicate. It can be done but often takes a long time depending on the amount of flukes in the liver. If you look at forums on the Internet people taking antihelmintic drugs have found that when clearing flukes they passed several hundred flukes every day in their stools.

There are many blogs (such as parasite drug forum) about liver fluke on the Internet where people share their experiences of taking multiple antihelmintic drugs and rotating them until they clear all the flukes.

Brand names of drugs used include:

- Egaten (Triclabendazole)
- Praziquantel
- Albendazole also Valbazen, which is the animal liquid form and is much cheaper
- Vermox (mebendazole)
- Yomesan (niclosamide)

Hydatid cysts of the liver

In humans hydatid disease is caused by the larvae of a flat tapeworm called Echinococcus granulosus. This parasitic infection occurs worldwide and is endemic in some countries such as Australia and the Middle East, especially in sheep farming areas.

Hydatid disease is a serious and potentially fatal condition, which may remain hidden in the body for many years.

How can humans become infected with this tapeworm?

Contact with dog feces or hair infected with the tapeworm eggs or contaminated vegetables cause hydatid disease in humans. The eggs may stick to the animal's hair or contaminate the vegetable garden. The eggs are highly resistant to the environment and can remain alive for months. Human infection does not occur from eating infected offal. Hydatid disease is not contagious and is not passed by person-to-person contact.

Life cycle of a tapeworm

The life cycle of the tapeworm alternates between herbivores and carnivores — (typically sheep, foxes and dogs). Humans are an accidental intermediate host and become an end point in the tapeworm's lifecycle.

The sheep ingests the eggs which hatch in the sheep's intestine and travel to the liver where the hydatid cyst develops. When a dog eats the sheep's organs containing the hydatid cyst, the dog becomes infected and passes eggs out in their feces. Cows and sheep become infected by eating the grass contaminated by dog feces. Other animals that may be infected include pigs, cattle, goats, horses, camels, wombats, wallabies and kangaroos. The grazing animal eats dog, fox or dingo feces infected with tapeworm eggs. Eventually the animal's organs (such as the liver, brain or lungs) grow watery sacs called hydatid cysts. These cysts contain around 40 tapeworm heads and a mature cyst may contain several million such heads.

Symptoms of Hydatid Disease

The symptoms of hydatid disease vary according to which body organs are infected. The most commonly infected organ is the liver, but the brain, kidneys and lungs are sometimes affected. In humans, the slow growing cysts are localized in the liver (in 75% of cases), the lungs (in 5-15% of cases) and other organs in the body such as the spleen, brain, heart and kidneys (in 10-20% of cases). The cysts are usually filled with a clear fluid called hydatid fluid and are spherical and usually consist of one compartment.

Symptoms can occur a long time after infection and sometimes many years later, but there may be no symptoms at all. If they occur, symptoms may include:

- Weight loss
- A swollen and bloated abdomen
- Anaemia
- Fatigue
- Cough and blood or liquid from a ruptured cyst – may be coughed up
- Jaundice – pressure from a growing cyst may obstruct the bile ducts
- Sometimes, a lack of vitamins can be caused in the host by the very high demand of the parasite to grow

If the cysts were to rupture while in the body, during surgical removal of the cysts or by some kind of trauma to the body, the patient would most likely go into a type of shock called anaphylaxis which leads to high fever, severe itching, hives, swelling (edema) of the lips and eyelids, shortness of breath, wheezing and sneezing.

Hydatid disease can be fatal without emergency medical treatment.

How is Hydatid disease diagnosed?

- By a thorough medical history and physical examination
- Imaging tests such as chest X-rays, ultrasound and CT or MRI scans
- Examination of blood, urine, sputum and feces
- Blood tests for antibodies to the cysts

Treatment of Hydatid Disease

The standard form of treatment is surgical removal of the cysts combined with drugs such as albendazole and/or mebendazole before surgery and for 8 weeks after surgery to clear up any spilled hydatid fluid containing live tapeworm components.

One of the risks of surgery is that a hydatid cyst may rupture and spread tapeworm heads throughout the patient's body. This risk is mitigated by prescribing high doses of the drug albendazole with the surgery, which helps to destroy any remaining tapeworm heads. Unfortunately the risk of recurrence of hydatid disease is high and around 30% of patients treated for hydatid disease develop the condition again and need repeat treatment.

If there are cysts in multiple organs or tissues, or the cysts are in dangerous places in the body, surgery may be too difficult and dangerous and in these cases drugs (Albendazole or Mebendazole) and/or PAIR (puncture-aspiration-injection-reaspiration) become the only possible treatment.

PAIR is a minimally invasive procedure that uses three steps:

- Puncture and needle aspiration of the cyst
- Injection of a scolicidal solution for 20-30 minutes
- Cyst-re-aspiration and final irrigation

When PAIR is performed patients take albendazole or mebendazole from 7 days before the procedure until 28 days after the procedure.

There is currently research into a new treatment called Percutaneous Thermal Ablation (PTA) of the germinal layer in the cyst by means of a radiofrequency ablation device. This form of treatment is still new and requires much more testing before being widely recommended.

Preventing infection with the Hydatid Tapeworm

There is a huge need for health education programs, improved water sanitation and better standards of hygiene.

Humans can become infected with echinococcus eggs via touching contaminated soil, animal feces and animal hair. It is also important to intervene at certain stages of the tape worm's life cycle, especially the infection of hosts (especially domestic dogs) living with or near humans.

Effective interventions include regular de-worming of dogs and vaccinating dogs and other livestock, such as sheep, that also act as hosts for the tapeworm.

Preventative suggestions include:

- Regular preventive de-worming of dogs. It is important to control tapeworm infection in domestic dogs. Infected dogs usually don't have any symptoms and appear healthy.
- Dispose of your dog's faeces carefully and wear rubber gloves. Wash your hands thoroughly after disposing of dog droppings.
- Always wash your hands with plenty of soap and water after touching your dog. Wash hands before eating and drinking and after gardening or handling animals.
- Never feed offal (either raw or cooked) to your dog.
- Take your dog to the vet for treatment with anti-tapeworm medication if you suspect an infection in your dog.
- If your dog has a proven infection, incinerate or bury deeply all dog feces until a cure is pronounced. Clean and disinfect the kennel and surrounding living area.
- Be especially vigilant if you are a sheep or cattle farmer and prevent your dogs from eating carcasses.
- Do not allow your dog to roam when holidaying in country areas.
- If you grow your own vegetables, fence your vegetable gardens to ensure that domestic and wild animals do not defecate on the soil.

Currently there are no human vaccines against any form of echinococcosis. However, there are studies being conducted for an effective human vaccine against echinococcosis.

Gallbladder conditions during pregnancy

It is common knowledge that pregnancy can be the initial trigger for a gallbladder problem or can aggravate a pre-existing gallbladder condition. Sometimes a gallbladder problem can worsen after a woman gives birth and this is more common with a caesarian delivery.

The main reason that gallbladder problems are more common in women than men is because women have much higher levels of estrogen in their body than men

Estrogen promotes a higher concentration of cholesterol to be secreted into the bile, which then enters the gallbladder. Too much cholesterol in the bile makes it thicker and prone to developing sludge and eventually stones. The sky high levels of estrogen during pregnancy can significantly aggravate this situation.

If gallbladder disease causes an obstruction to the flow of bile in pregnancy, this condition is called cholestasis of pregnancy. It occurs in roughly one in one thousand pregnancies and is most common in the third trimester of pregnancy, when hormone levels are at their peak. The condition is more common in women with a family history of gallbladder disease, older women (older than 35 years) and in women who have had several children.

Cholestasis just means obstruction to the normal flow of bile.

Pregnancy hormones affect gallbladder function, resulting in slowing or stopping the flow of bile. If the bile flow is stopped or slowed down, this causes a build up of bile acids in the liver which can spill into the bloodstream. This means there will be too much bilirubin in the bloodstream, which can cause jaundice and other symptoms.

The most common symptoms of cholestasis in pregnancy are:

- Itching, especially of the hands and feet
- Nausea
- Loss of appetite

- Light (tan) colored stool
- Dark colored urine
- Jaundice (yellowing of the eyes and skin)
- Pain or discomfort in the right upper quadrant of the abdomen

Does cholestasis of pregnancy harm the baby?

Cholestasis of pregnancy places stress on the fetus' liver and can result in premature delivery or stillbirth.

The condition can result in abnormally high levels of bile salt in the blood of the fetus. Luckily, cholestasis of pregnancy is most common in the third trimester, because if the lungs of the fetus have developed adequately, labour may be induced prematurely in order to save the fetus.

The treatment plan we have outlined in chapter two can be safely followed by most pregnant women, although we ask you to be guided by your own doctor. It is safe to make the diet changes we suggest, but please avoid using any herbs while pregnant.

Medication to decrease the concentration of bile acids such as ursodeoxycholic acid (Ursofalk) is safe and effective in pregnancy and it is the main remedy used by doctors for cholestasis of pregnancy. The daily dose used is between 600 mg and 2000 mg of ursodeoxycholic acid. It is generally very effective for reducing itching, as well as blood levels of bilirubin, bile acid and ALT liver enzyme levels. [23.] This is the same medication that anyone wishing to dissolve gallstones can take and we have covered it in detail on page 90.

Chapter
Eleven

How to live well without a gallbladder:

Important information for those who have had their gallbladder removed

Thousands of people have their gallbladder removed each day; it is one of the most commonly performed surgical procedures.

Your doctor probably told you that your gallbladder is not necessary and you can survive perfectly fine without it. That is partly true; yes you can survive without a gallbladder but you cannot thrive unless you take particularly good care of your liver and digestive system.

Your doctor may have told you that once you get your gallbladder removed, you'll be able to "eat whatever you like" and no longer experience pain or discomfort. Perhaps that turned out not to be true. Worse still, a large number of people are left with even worse symptoms than before they lost their gallbladder - chronic diarrhea, indigestion and irritable bowel syndrome.

What happens when you don't have a gallbladder?

Your liver continues to manufacture bile, but there is no longer a place to store it or concentrate it. Therefore bile continually slowly trickles into the intestines.

If you eat a fatty meal, you will not be able to secrete a large enough amount of bile into your intestines, therefore the fat will be poorly digested. This means many people experience diarrhea, bloating, nausea or indigestion after eating fat.

Not digesting fat well means you will not be able to absorb essential fatty acids, including omega 3 and omega 6 fats

It also means you'll have a hard time absorbing fat soluble vitamins such as vitamins D, E, A and K. A lot of the antioxidants in vegetables are fat soluble: lycopene, lutein and carotenoids are all fat soluble.

If you don't produce adequate bile, you will not be adequately absorbing these life saving compounds from foods.

If you take any of the above mentioned nutrients in supplement form, without sufficient bile you will sadly not absorb them well.

Post cholecystectomy syndrome

- Your gallbladder is gone but all your problems are still here

Post cholecystectomy syndrome is the term used to describe the presence of abdominal symptoms after surgical removal of the gallbladder.

It is thought to occur in between five and 40 percent of patients who have had their gallbladder removed. [24.] Symptoms include persistent right upper abdominal pain, diarrhea, nausea, flatulence and abdominal bloating.

Firstly it is important to rule out a serious medical problem such as post surgical adhesions, injury to the liver or a bile duct during surgery, or a trapped stone within a bile duct. Unfortunately, the usual scenario is that these factors have been ruled out, yet the patient continues to experience a great deal of pain or discomfort.

Some people experience chronic constipation as a result of losing their gallbladder, as bile normally has a gentle laxative effect and less bile now enters the small intestine. Other people experience chronic diarrhea since having their gallbladder removed because the continual trickle of bile acids into the intestines irritates the intestinal lining.

The conventional medical treatment is to give the patient the drug cholestyramine which impairs the absorption of bile acids; it binds to them and takes them out of the body in the stool. However cholestyramine also impairs the absorption of all fat soluble nutrients such as vitamins, essential fatty acids and antioxidants, so it is not a good long term solution.

We have found that food allergy or intolerance is the single greatest cause of continual pain, discomfort and digestive problems following cholecystectomy.

Food sensitivity caused the original gallbladder problem, therefore removing the gallbladder wasn't the right solution; it just created a whole new set of problems. So stop eating the foods that caused your original problem.

Even without a gallbladder, you can still form stones

That's right, the stones just won't be in your gallbladder; they can form inside your common bile duct, or inside the hepatic ducts inside your liver. Stones in those locations are much more difficult to treat and they can create just as much pain as stones within the gallbladder. Stones in the common bile duct can quickly become infected and require urgent medical treatment. Stones within the bile ducts inside the liver can cause inflammation and damage to liver cells and increase the risk of liver cysts.

That means even if your gallbladder has been removed, you are not in the clear

You still need to follow each of the recommendations in chapter two if you want to avoid future health problems. It is also crucial to remember that you developed gallstones in the first place for a reason; several reasons probably. Just removing the storage sac for bile does not undo all the problems that caused the gallstones in the first place.

Strategies for maintaining good health without a gallbladder

People who don't have a gallbladder are at increased risk of various health problems. Here are some ways to avoid them.

- Take a good quality liver tonic that contains the herbs St Mary's thistle and dandelion. These herbs improve the ability of your liver to produce bile and help to keep the bile moving through your liver and bile ducts. These herbs should help to make you feel more comfortable after a meal, and should reduce the risk of stones forming inside your liver.

  People who have had their gallbladder removed are at greater risk of developing a fatty liver and these herbs help to reduce that risk also.

- Take an ox bile supplement. **This is the single most important recommendation for anyone who has lost their gallbladder.**

  A lack of bile can produce symptoms such as bloating and indigestion after meals, light colored stools, diarrhea or constipation, fatigue after meals and nutrient deficiencies. Taking a good quality ox bile supplement with each meal is wonderful for completely eliminating these symptoms in most individuals. Bile is absolutely critical for normal fat digestion because it breaks down large fat globules into tiny ones so that digestive enzymes can work on them and break them down.

Without sufficient bile, you will not be absorbing essential fatty acids, fat soluble vitamins or antioxidants properly

If you take these nutrients in supplement form, you will not be getting your money's worth if you have insufficient bile in your digestive tract. An ox bile supplement is an inexpensive way to ensure proper fat digestion and you should take one capsule with each meal for the rest of your life. You may need to take a digestive enzymes supplement as well if you do not experience adequate improvements with ox bile alone. For more information see www. liverdoctor.com

- Eat some good fats and avoid the bad fats. Your doctor may have recommended you follow a low fat diet after having your gallbladder removed. This is not necessary and in fact it is harmful. Your body desperately needs good fats and we recommend you include moderate quantities of extra virgin olive oil, avocados, coconut milk and oil, nuts and seeds in your diet, assuming you don't have an allergy to any of these foods. You should be able to handle moderate amounts of animal fats too, such as pastured (grass fed) butter, lard, suet and tallow.

- You may need a vitamin D3 supplement. People with compromised liver or digestive function are often vitamin D deficient. Exposure of your skin to the sun's UVB rays enables your body to manufacture vitamin D. However, this process occurs in your liver and kidneys. People with a sluggish or overworked liver often do not manufacture vitamin D adequately. Therefore it's a good idea to get a blood test and take a supplement if necessary.

  For optimal health your blood vitamin D level should be between 40 and 60 ng/mL. Taking 5000 IU of vitamin D3 is a safe and effective dose for most people, but it's best to be guided by your own doctor.

- Include some bitter and sour foods in your diet. They should help to improve your digestion and make it easier to tolerate good fats in your diet. Suitable bitter and sour foods include lemons, limes, radicchio lettuce, chicory, endive and dandelion leaves. These leaves are fairly easy to grow at home if you are lucky enough to have your own veggie patch.

- Find out if you have a food allergy or sensitivity. If you still experience pain or digestive problems after having your gallbladder removed, there is a very good chance you are eating foods your body considers harmful. The biggest culprits are dairy products, gluten, eggs, onions, pork, corn and soy. So for starters, avoid those foods and see if you feel any better. You may need the help of a naturopath or nutritionist to help you identify your food sensitivities.

- Increase your liver's ability to manufacture glutathione by taking a selenium supplement and a supplement of N-acetyl cysteine (NAC). Glutathione is the body's most powerful antioxidant and it helps to improve your liver's detoxification abilities. Bile is an important excretion route of toxins from the body. If you would like more information, please call us on 1888 755 4837 and speak to one of our nutritional advisors.

If you follow our suggestions, you can enjoy excellent health despite no longer having your gallbladder.

Chapter Twelve

Recipes and Food Ideas

In this chapter you will find some gallbladder friendly recipes as well as a handy shopping list which should help when stocking your pantry.

Super Quick Shopping List

- Vegetables - non starchy: celery, endive, radishes, lettuce, carrots, tomatoes, leek, onions, garlic
  - starchy: sweet potato, turnip, etc.
  - dark leafy greens: spinach, watercress, mustard greens, Asian greens, beets and beet leaves, etc.
- Fruit - berries, apples, grapes, plums, oranges, lemons, limes and avocado
- Raw nuts and seeds - raw almonds, raw cashews, pine nuts, sunflower seeds, pepitas and chia seeds
- Red meat - preferably grass fed
- Canned salmon, tuna, sardines, mackeral and trout
- Fresh seafood - fish, lobster, crab, prawns and calamari
- Free range chicken
- Cold pressed oils - extra virgin olive, macadamia, coconut or avocado
- Apple cider vinegar
- Fresh herbs - parsley, mint, basil, cilantro, etc.
- Tahini
- Herbal teas - peppermint, lemongrass, ginger or green tea

Raw vegetable juice for the gallbladder

Serves 1

Drink this vegetable juice regularly, whether you decide to do a gallbladder flush or not. Try to drink one glass of this juice every day, or as often as possible.

Ingredients	1 large beet
	8 large beet leaves
	8 chicory or endive leaves
	2 stalks celery
	¼ red onion
	1 large carrot
	2 red radishes
	1 small apple
Method	Pass all ingredients through a juice extractor and drink.
	Sometimes it is hard to find fresh beet leaves. The beet may look good but the leaves are wilted and completely dead. You may also have difficulty finding chicory or endive. Beet leaves are particularly beneficial for the gallbladder.
	Chicory and endive are very bitter and all bitter foods stimulate the release of bile from the gallbladder. This helps to prevent bile stagnation in the gallbladder.

Super smoothie

Serves 1

Coconut oil is high in medium chain triglycerides, which are a type of fat that does not require bile for digestion. The fats in coconut oil are taken straight to the liver and used for energy.

Ingredients

1 cup coconut, hemp or other non-dairy milk

2 teaspoons organic coconut oil

½ cup fresh or frozen blueberries

1 tablespoon dried goji berries

1 tablespoon chia seeds

1 large handful spinach, kale or other dark green leaves

Method

Soak the goji berries in ¼ cup water for several hours to soften them. Place all ingredients, including the water the goji berries have been soaked in into a blender and process until smooth.

You can enjoy this smoothie for breakfast or as a snack.

Green salad dressing

This is really a cross between a salad dressing and a pesto. We like to use it as a salad dressing.

Ingredients

2 large handfuls fresh parsley

1 large handful fresh mint leaves

½ cup extra virgin olive oil or avocado oil

Juice and zest of one lime

2 tablespoons apple cider vinegar

Method

Place all ingredients into a powerful blender and process until smooth. Use to dress any salad.

Serves 2

This soup is rich in those vegetables specifically beneficial for your liver and gallbladder. Try and include them as often as possible in your diet. Remember that variety is the spice of life so don't only use them in soup, you can always steam them and drizzle with olive oil and lemon juice or you could add them to stews or casseroles.

Ingredients
1 leek, washed thoroughly and sliced

2 teaspoons organic coconut oil

27 oz water or vegetable stock, or water flavored with ½ teaspoon Herbamare (available in supermarkets)

1 bunch endive or chicory, chopped

1 broccoli floret, chopped

Leaves from one bunch of beets

2 medium zucchinis, chopped

Method
Heat the coconut oil gently in a large pot and add the chopped leek. Saute for 3 to 4 minutes, until softened. Add all remaining ingredients, bring to the boil and then reduce heat to a gentle simmer. Cook until all vegetables are softened.

You can puree the soup in a blender or serve it chunky.

This soup can be served on its own as an entree but if having it as a meal, please add some cooked chicken or fish as a source of protein.

Raw beet salad for the gallbladder

Serves 2 as a side salad

This is a delicious salad full of healthy foods for your gallbladder. Try to eat it several times a week.

Ingredients	2 beets, peeled and grated medium fine
	1 medium apple, grated coarsely
	2 tablespoons fresh lemon juice
	1 tablespoon apple cider vinegar
	2 tablespoons extra virgin olive oil
	1 tablespoon chia seeds (*put them in just before serving*)
Method	Combine grated beets and apple together in a bowl. Combine lemon juice, vinegar and oil together in a small bowl and whisk together well. Pour dressing over salad and toss well. Sprinkle chia seeds into salad and serve.

Guacamole

Avocados are high in good monounsaturated fats. When eaten in moderate quantities they are easy to digest and don't place a strain on the liver or gallbladder.

Ingredients	Flesh from 2 ripe avocados
	Juice of one lime
	¼ cup finely chopped cilantro
	1 small finely diced chilli (optional)
	Sea salt and pepper to taste
Method	You can either mash all the ingredients together well with a fork, or puree them in a food processor. Serve as a snack with raw vegetables or dollop over a

Serves 4

Ingredients

1 pound chicken thighs

1 tablespoon olive or macadamia nut oil

¼ cup fresh lime juice

¼ cup Dijon mustard

¼ cup fresh cilantro, finely chopped

1 teaspoon turmeric powder

½ teaspoon each of salt and pepper

Method

Place all ingredients except chicken into a food processor and blend until combined and smooth.

Place the chicken thighs into a baking dish. Pour the mustard mixture over the chicken, making sure all parts of the chicken are well covered.

Cover the dish and place in the refrigerator overnight.

The next day, bake in a 350 degree Fahrenheit oven for approximately 20 minutes, or until cooked.

Serve with a salad or cooked vegetables.

Lemon and rosemary chicken

Serves 4

Ingredients

1 pound chicken thighs

¼ cup fresh lemon juice

1 teaspoon finely grated lemon zest

2 tablespoons olive oil

1 clove garlic, crushed

2 tablespoons finely chopped fresh rosemary leaves

1 tablespoon finely chopped fresh parsley leaves

½ teaspoon salt

Method

Combine all ingredients except chicken together in a bowl and whisk until well combined.

Place chicken into a baking dish and pour marinade on top, making sure all parts of the chicken are well covered.

Cover the baking dish and place in the fridge overnight.

The next day, bake in a 350 degree Fahrenheit oven for approximately 20 minutes, or until cooked.

Serve with a salad or cooked vegetables.

salmon with tomatoes and basil

Ingredients

½ pound fresh salmon fillets

1 cup cherry tomatoes, sliced in half

2 cloves garlic, crushed

½ small red onion, very finely sliced

2 teaspoons apple cider vinegar

1 tablespoon olive oil

¼ cup fresh basil leaves, torn

½ teaspoon salt

Method

Preheat the oven to 300 degrees Fahrenheit.

Wash the salmon fillets and pat them dry with paper towels. Place the salmon into a baking dish. Arrange sliced tomatoes, onion, garlic and basil leaves on top.

Drizzle olive oil and vinegar over the top, cover the baking dish and bake in the oven for approximately 15 minutes, or until done to your liking.

Serve with a salad or cooked vegetables.

Lamb chops with rosemary and garlic

Serves 4

Ingredients

1.4 pound rack of lamb

6 cloves of garlic, finely chopped

¼ cup fresh rosemary leaves, finely chopped

1 teaspoon ground cumin

2 tablespoons coconut oil

½ teaspoon each of salt and pepper

Method

Preheat the oven to 400 degrees Fahrenheit. Saute the rosemary and garlic in one teaspoon of coconut oil until softened.

Cut the rack of lamb into individual chops. Pat them dry with a paper towel.

Sprinkle salt and pepper over the chops. Heat the remaining coconut oil in a skillet over medium heat and sear the chops for 2 minutes on each side.

Transfer the chops to a baking dish, sprinkle the rosemary and cumin over them and bake in the oven until cooked to your liking.

Serve with a salad or cooked vegetables.

Healthier mashed potato

Ingredients
2 medium sweet potatoes, peeled and chopped roughly

1 pound carrots, peeled and chopped

1 tablespoon organic coconut oil, melted

A sprinkle of sea salt or Herbamare

Method
Preheat the oven to 425 degrees F.

Arrange all ingredients on a lined or greased baking tray and roast in the oven until very soft and lightly browned. You may need to toss them around a couple of times while cooking.

Once the vegetables are cooked, place them into a food processor or blender with the following ingredients:

2 teaspoons organic coconut oil

½ teaspoon paprika

½ teaspoon salt

A sprinkle of black pepper

You may need a teaspoon or so of water or coconut milk

Blend the whole mixture together until smooth and then serve.

Glossary

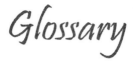

Acalculous cholecystitis
Inflammation of the gallbladder with no gallstones inside it. Acalculous means without stones.

Bile
Manufactured in the liver from a combination of cholesterol, bilirubin, bile acids, lecithin and waste products. Stored in the gallbladder and required for fat digestion.

Biliary dyskinesia
Refers to abnormal movement and flow of bile through the biliary system. It is a motility disorder and can be caused by inefficient gallbladder contractions, dysfunction of the sphincter of Oddi or abnormal contractions of the biliary ducts. The condition can produce pain and discomfort without the presence of gallstones.

Bilirubin
A component of bile which is made in the liver from worn out old red blood cells.

Cholagogue
A substance that promotes contraction of the gallbladder and release of bile into the small intestine. Some herbs and foods have cholagogue actions.

Cholangiogram
A type of X ray where a dye is injected into the bile duct to watch its course and check for the presence of stones or blockages in the bile ducts.

Cholangitis
Inflammation of a bile duct.

Cholecystectomy
Surgical removal of the gallbladder.

Cholecystitis
Inflammation of the gallbladder.

Cholecystokinin (CCK)
A hormone made by the cells of the small intestine which travels to the gallbladder and stimulates it to contract. The presence of food, and especially fat in the small intestine stimulates release of CCK.

Choledocholithiasis
The presence of gallstones in the common bile duct.

Cholelithiasis
The presence of gallstones in the gallbladder.

Choleretic
A substance that increases the production of bile in the liver. Some herbs and foods have choleretic actions.

Cholestasis
Disruption (stasis) to the normal flow of bile. May be caused by a blockage of a bile duct and can lead to elevated levels of bilirubin in the blood, producing jaundice.

Jaundice
Elevated bilirubin in the bloodstream, caused by a liver or gallbladder problem. The high level of bilirubin in the blood causes yellowing of the whites of the eyes and skin.

Post cholecystectomy syndrome
Pain and other symptoms present after surgery to remove the gallbladder.

References

1. British Journal of General Practice 2004; 54:574-79

2. Paumgartner G, Sauerbruch T: Gallstones: pathogenesis. Lancet 338 :1117– 1121,1991

3. Hayes KC, Livingston A, Trautwein EA: Dietary impact on biliary lipids and gallstones. Annu Rev Nutr12 :299– 326,1992

4. Is bile flow reduced in patients with hypothyroidism? Surgery 2003 Mar; 133():288-93

5. Chen DF, et al. H pylori are associated with chronic cholecystitis. World J Gastroenterol 2007 Feb 21;13(7):1119-22.

6. R. W. L. Leong, J. J. Y. Sung. Helicobacter species and hepatobiliary diseases. Alimentary Pharmacology & Therapeutics Volume 16, Issue 6, pages 1037–1045, June 2002

7. C. J. Tsai, et al. Long term effect of magnesium consumption on the risk of symptomatic gallstone disease among men. The American Journal Of Gastroenterology. Feb 2008, volume 103, issue 2, pages 375-382

8. Leitzmann MF, Willett WC, Rimm EB, et al. A prospective study of coffee consumption and the risk of symptomatic gallstone disease in men. JAMA 1999;281:2106-2112

9. Leitzmann MF, Stampfer MJ, Willett WC, et al. Coffee intake is associated with lower risk of symptomatic gallstone disease in women. Gastroenterology 2002;123:1823-1830.

10. Sreedevi Koppisetti et al. Reactive Oxygen Species and the Hypomotility of the Gall Bladder as Targets for the Treatment of Gallstones with Melatonin: A Review. Digestive Diseases and Sciences October 2008, Volume 53, Issue 10, pp 2592-2603

11. Moerman CJ, Smeets FW, Kromhout D: Dietary risk factors for clinically diagnosed gallstones in middle-aged men. A 25-year follow-up study (the Zutphen Study). Ann Epidemiol4 :248– 254,1994

12. Jeff S. Volek, Stephen D. Phinney. The Art and Science of Low

Carbohydrate Living. 2011 Beyond Obesity LLC

13. Maton PN, Selden AC, Fitzpatrick ML, Chadwick VS. Defective gallbladder emptying and cholecystokinin release in celiac disease. Reversal by gluten-free diet. Gastroenterology 1985;88:391-396

14. Breneman JC. Allergy elimination diet as the most effective gallbladder diet. Ann Allergy 1968;26:83-87

15. Capper WM, Butler TJ, Kilby JO, Gibson MJ. Gallstones, gastric secretion and flatulent dyspepsia. Lancet 1967;1:413-415

16. Schaefer O: When the Eskimo come to town. Nutr Today8 :16 ,1971

17. Berr F, Holl J, Jungst D, Fischer S, Richter WO, Seifferth B, Paumgartner G: Dietary n-3 polyunsaturated fatty acids decrease biliary cholesterol saturation in gallstone disease. Hepatology16 :960– 967,1992

18. Kaude JV, The width of the common bile duct in relation to age and stone disease. An ultrasonographic study. Eur J Radiol. 1983 May;3(2):115-7

19. Sies CW, Brooker J. Could these be gallstones? Lancet 2005;365:1388

20. British Journal of General Practice 2004; 54:574-79

21. Am J Gastroenterology 92:132-38, 1997

22. Kumar S, et al Infection as a risk factor for gallbladder cancer. J Surg Oncol. 2006 Jun 15;93(8):633-9.

23. Glantz A, et al. Intrahepatic cholestasis of pregnancy: a randomized controlled trial comparing dexamethasone and ursodeoxycholic acid. Hepatology Dec 2005;42(6):1399-405

24. Glasgow RE, Mulvihill SJ (2010). Treatment of gallstone disease. In M Feldman et al., eds., Sleisenger and Fordtran's Gastrointestinal and Liver Disease, 9th ed., vol. 1, pp. 1121-1138. Philadelphia: Saunders.

Index

globe artichoke - 24, 28-29, 49, 68-69, 96

gluten - 7, 14, 32, 42-44, 45-47, 49, 67-68, 84, 93, 96, 111

glycine - 34, 69, 72

HIDA scan - 43, 79-80, 92

hydatid cysts - 101

hypochlorhydria - 14, 43, 48

hypothyroidism - 14, 31

insulin resistance (also see syndrome X) - 14, 35, 38

jaundice - 60, 82, 92, 95, 97, 102, 105-106, 124

liver - 7-11, 12-15, 17, 20, 22-23, 26-31, 36, 39-43, 47, 53, 56, 60, 64, 69-74, 79-84, 87, 89-90, 95-102, 105-112, 115-117, 123-124

liver fluke - 96-100

magnesium - 33, 35-36, 57, 63, 67, 69

malic acid - 36-37, 59, 63, 69

meal plan - 50

melatonin - 37-38

milk - 32, 46-47, 49-50, 52, 69, 111, 115, 122

milk thistle (also see St Mary's thistle) - 27

n-acetyl cysteine - 36, 96, 112

ox bile - 34-35, 48, 54, 67, 69, 110-111

pancreatitis - 83, 85, 92

peppermint - 29, 33, 57, 67, 113

porcelain gallbladder - 11, 95

pregnancy - 13-14, 82, 105-106

primary biliary cirrhosis - 5, 11, 83, 89, 95

sclerosing cholangitis - 11, 83, 95

selenium - 36, 42, 63, 93-94, 96, 112

St Mary's thistle - 27-28, 69, 96, 110

syndrome x - 14, 35, 37-38

tapeworm - 101, 103-104

taurine - 34, 63, 69, 72, 96

ultrasound - 11, 60, 65, 79, 87-89, 93, 95, 98-99, 102

ursodeoxycholic acid - 35, 89, 95, 106

vitamin C - 10, 33, 35, 42, 69